The Therapist's Ultimate Solution Book

NORTON PROFESSIONAL BOOKS

THE THERAPIST'S ULTIMATE SOLUTION BOOK

*Essential Strategies, Tips & Tools
to Empower Your Clients*

Judith Belmont

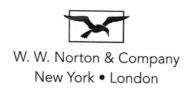

W. W. Norton & Company
New York • London

For information about permission to reproduce selections from this book, write to
Permissions, W. W. Norton & Company, Inc., 500 Fifth Avenue, New York, NY 10110

For information about special discounts for bulk purchases, please contact
W. W. Norton Special Sales at specialsales@wwnorton.com or 800-233-4830

Manufacturing by Courier Westford
Production manager: Christine Critelli

Library of Congress Cataloging-in-Publication Data

Belmont, Judith.
 The therapist's ultimate solution book : essential strategies, tips & tools
to empower your clients / Judith Belmont. — First edition.
     pages cm. — (A norton professional book)
 Includes bibliographical references and index.
 ISBN 978-0-393-70988-9 (hardcover)
 1. Psychotherapy. 2. Self-help techniques. 3. Psychotherapist and
patient. I. Title.
   RC480.B358 2015
   616.89'14—dc23
       2014046222

ISBN: 978-0-393-70988-9

W. W. Norton & Company, Inc., 500 Fifth Avenue, New York, N.Y. 10110
www.wwnorton.com
W. W. Norton & Company Ltd., Castle House, 75/76 Wells Street, London W1T 3QT

1 2 3 4 5 6 7 8 9 0

Contents

Contents

Contents

Contents

Acknowledgments

I am grateful for the many clients and colleagues who over the years have helped shape my interest in solution-oriented psychological treatment.

Thanks to the talented Norton staff, especially editors Andrea Costella Dawson and Ben Yarling for their expert guidance in developing this book, as well as copy editor Rachel Keith. Thanks also to Katie Moyer, assistant managing editor, and Kevin Olsen, marketing manager.

Thanks most of all to my husband, Don, for his consistent support and editorial assistance in bringing this book to fruition.

The Therapist's Ultimate Solution Book

Introduction

As clinicians, we work in all types of settings and deal with a wide variety of clients. No matter what setting we work in as clinicians, however, there are certain common denominators across the board. One is that our clients seek help for their problems, and they look to us to provide the expertise to help unlock solutions. Second, as clinicians we have the responsibility to educate ourselves so that we can teach our clients practical life skills. Just as a construction worker needs a well-supplied toolbox to build anything substantial, therapists equipped with the right combination of tools in their therapeutic toolbox will be able to tailor treatment to address almost any of their clients' needs and life challenges. Solution-oriented clinicians who learn an array of targeted, easy-to-learn and easy-to-teach psychoeducational strategies will be more flexible and more adept at treating the range of symptoms their clients present.

Clients generally come to therapy *wanting to* change, but they often have no inherent knowledge of *how to* change. By offering them life-skills tools, clinicians can help them make long-standing life changes. These strategies are by no means one-size-fits-all. This book provides therapists with a wide selection of tools, such as behavioral logs, worksheets, handouts, activities, visualizations, metaphors, and mini-lessons, to fit the array of client needs.

The Therapist as Teacher: Psychoeducation in Solution-Oriented Treatment

The role of the therapist is not just to listen, support, and offer feedback and suggestions—it is also to teach!

The solution-oriented approach often entails giving clients general education on a topic before attempting to help them change and learn new skills. Just as a piano teacher can't expect a student to come to the initial lessons knowing how to read music notation, clinicians can't expect clients to come to therapy with the basic set of skills they need to make healthy life changes. Clients need knowledge, education, and proven strategies to practice any newly acquired skills. For example, clients may never have learned the basics of assertive communication, and may not be able to differentiate aggressive from assertive statements. Therefore, they may find themselves getting into problematic relationships and have no clue about how to get out of them. Or they may never have learned how to separate their thoughts from their feelings, and therefore lack the knowledge of how to tell them apart, leading to symptoms of crippling anxiety or depression. The resource materials in this book provide clients with many opportunities to practice the skills offered in each chapter. Furthermore, since learning new skills requires practice, making it a habit to complete homework assignments between sessions is vital to the effectiveness of any modern psychotherapy treatment. After all, how effective would it be to learn to ride a bike or repair cars if you learned about them theoretically without a lot of practice? You don't learn by talking; you learn by *doing*.

Let's use the analogy of the piano student again. After the student comes to the initial lessons and is introduced to the basics of reading notes and scales, he or she needs to practice *between* lessons. Just as the piano student practices music scales, the therapy client needs to practice the skills learned in session. For both piano student and client, showing up for weekly sessions without practicing in between will make for very limited progress. We wouldn't expect the piano student to catch on to concepts newly learned just by showing up for scheduled appointments, nor should we expect that of our clients. Only after the fundamental skills are mastered with a lot of practice will the piano student or the therapy client learn to make beautiful music, literally and figuratively. This focus on homework is a cornerstone of most current counseling approaches. Cognitive Behavior Therapy, Dialectical Behavioral Therapy, and other modern approaches use self-help materials for between-session skill building. Drs. Aaron and Judith Beck, for example, emphasize the importance of practice and homework in Cognitive Behavior Therapy to help clients increase their effectiveness in helping themselves.

A common misperception about the psychoeducational approach is that teaching clients is too dogmatic and amounts to telling them what to do or how to be. To the contrary, offering handouts, worksheets, activities, and structured exercises to clients does not take their control away. Rather, it helps them develop skills to take control of their lives and stop giving so much control to others! It teaches them new solutions to old problems as well as strategies to generate new ways of coping. After all, tools are meaningless unless you know how to use them. Thus, teaching does not mean taking away clients' autonomy; it offers choices when they don't know alternatives. This proactive approach empowers clients with tools for life and helps them deal with change constructively.

As Confucius so aptly said, "Teach me and I will forget, show me and I will remember, involve me and I will understand." Psychoeducation does, however, have its limits. Although the tools presented can certainly serve as helpful coping strategies, there are times that behavior is so ingrained that feelings and thoughts are extremely resistant to treatment. In these cases, treatment ideally takes place while the client is medically managed with more in-depth psychiatric care. Clients need to be ready both biologically and psychologically to make use of the tools given. Appreciating the need to work with psychiatric and medical professionals to help the client become ready to learn and heal is important in any effective treatment.

The Therapeutic Relationship: The Basis for Healthy Change

Action-oriented solutions to everyday problems won't work if you don't pay proper attention to establishing a baseline of security and mutual respect with your client. Techniques and life-skills strategies need a rich soil of therapeutic trust and safety to blossom. Psychological pioneer Carl Roger's emphasis on the importance of the nonjudgmental relationship, characterized by having "unconditional positive regard" for the client, needs to underlie any treatment for change. People will not change for the best if they don't feel their therapist is on their side or likes them. There is no substitute for true empathetic concern and an atmosphere of acceptance in forming a strong alliance in which clients can be free to grow and learn. This foundation is vital if you expect them to take risks and expand their comfort zones while performing their homework assignments. Only with a foundation of trust and empathy can clients feel safe to learn to help themselves. Even Rational Emotive Therapy founder Albert Ellis, with his very directive and blunt approach, emphasized the importance of the empathetic therapeutic relationship underlying any attempts to help clients change.

Solution-Oriented Treatment: Catching the Wave

Many of the treatment tools in this book would be considered examples of the second and third waves of psychotherapy. Cognitive Behavior Therapy is considered to represent the second wave of psychological intervention. Its pioneers include Albert Ellis, whose Rational Emotive Behavior Therapy (REBT) modality was the first formalized theory with a cognitive behavioral focus in the 1950s, setting the stage a decade later for Aaron Beck, who coined the term *Cognitive Behavior Therapy* (CBT).

The third wave of treatment incorporates the traditional cognitive approach while moving beyond it to include innovative therapeutic tools, for example, traditionally non-clinical treatments such as mindfulness and acceptance practices. These Eastern practices have become integrated with cognitive behavioral treatment in the new disciplines of today's psychological landscape. The best known are Dialectical Behavior Therapy (DBT), originated by Marsha Linehan; Acceptance and Commitment Therapy (ACT), founded by Steven Hayes; and Mindfulness-Based Cognitive Therapy (MBCT), an eight-week program spearheaded by Jon Kabat-Zinn that teaches depression and stress management, typically in medically based settings. All of these theories are psychoed-ucational in nature and rely heavily on experiential exercises and self-help materials that serve to educate as well as heal.

Third-wave cognitive behavior therapies are solution-oriented thera-pies, and I frequently refer to these as well as to various well-established CBT strategies throughout the book. My aim in writing this book is to offer "user-friendly," action-oriented strategies that clients can readily use to improve their coping skills in everyday life. Homework assignments, cognitive restructuring and acceptance practices, and mindfulness-based techniques are all characteristics of the innovative and experiential third wave of psychological treatment.

This third wave emerged from the awareness that traditional types of behavioral and cognitive behavior therapy could not reach many treatment-resistant populations, such as people with addictive person-alities, borderline and other personality disorders, and chronic mood disorders. To understand a little more about the third wave of treatment, it's helpful to first get an understanding of the first two waves of modern therapy. At the end of this section is a chart to help you differentiate the three waves of psychological treatment approaches.

The First Wave

The first wave of psychotherapy refers to the modality of Behavior Therapy, in which classical and operant-conditioning principles were applied to treating clinical problems. B. F. Skinner, Ivan Pavlov, and Joseph Wolpe, whose work spanned the late 1800s to mid-1900s, were all pioneers in the first wave. Observable behaviorism was a reaction to Freud's mentalistic concepts, which were not measurable. In Behavior Therapy, maladaptive actions are replaced through reinforcement and other conditioning techniques by more adaptive behaviors that the therapist facilitates in treatment. For example, to tackle everyday prob-lems, a system of reinforcements, such as the use of behavioral charting and various rewards for positive behaviors, might be used to "condi-tion" the client to have more adaptive responses and behaviors.

Whereas psychodynamic treatment relied on subjectivity, behavioral treatment using conditioning principles relied only on observable outcomes that could be objectively measured. The psychoanalytic treatment techniques of Freud, such as stream of consciousness, free association, dream interpretation, and transference, were replaced with attention to *cause and effect* and the principles of reinforcement. Underlying this drastic shift from psychoanalysis was the idea that insight was not the same as the cure, and that insight alone actually did little to cure most problems such as depression, anxiety, and panic.

Examples of techniques of the first wave include relaxation training, systematic desensitization, token economy, behavior modification, and biofeedback. Even though traditional behaviorism has been supplanted for the most part by cognitive behavioral and third-wave approaches, some treatment techniques from this discipline remain, designed to shape changes in people's behavior within educational, institutional, and treatment settings. Interestingly enough, there has been a resurgence of interest in relaxation and desensitization techniques in the third-wave approaches, tying behavioral approaches with the Eastern approaches of mindfulness and acceptance. You might say that the East and West have met, integrating the approaches of ancient wisdom with newer ones that are behavioral in orientation to treat many common psychological symptoms.

The Second Wave

The first wave set the stage for the second wave of behavioral treatment, which is the most widely adopted and empirically studied treatment in the world—cognitive behavior therapy, formally developed in the 1960s by Aaron Beck. It is by far the most rapidly growing psychological orientation throughout the world.

There have been many thousands of research studies done to support the effectiveness of Cognitive Behavior Therapy. CBT has been proven to be effective in the treatment of depression, anxiety, and other symptoms that result from chronic ruminative, obsessive, and persistent maladaptive patterns of thinking. CBT has in its origins the foundation of behavioral approaches to treatment, and departs from the traditional theories of conditioning by its focus on thoughts and feelings, notions which traditional behaviorists rejected as being too mentalistic and subjective. Interestingly enough, Ellis and Beck, the cognitive behavioral pioneers, were both trained psychoanalysts who found that psychoanalytic practice did not help their patients interpret events more accurately and did not offer solutions to many of the symptoms their clients presented. The underlying principle of the cognitive behavioral approach is that irrational and unhealthy thoughts lead to disturbing feelings, such as low self-esteem, depression, and anxiety. In turn, these disruptive and maladaptive feelings lead to unhealthy behaviors, such as social withdrawal, relationship conflicts, substance abuse, and other self-sabotaging behaviors.

With Ellis and Beck setting the foundation, other CBT therapists popularized the approach through various handbooks and self-help books using CBT practices. Perhaps the most widely read CBT expert is David Burns, who made CBT accessible to millions of readers in his best-selling books *Feeling Good: The New Mood Therapy* (1980), *Ten Days to Self Esteem* (1993a), and *The Feeling Good Handbook* (1999), among others. In fact, in the introduction to his *Feeling Good Handbook*, Burns cites his research on self-help bibliotherapy. He found that giving prospective patients waiting to begin therapy at his Philadelphia clinic a copy of his *Feeling Good Handbook* was much more effective than a placebo. In fact, once the patients using bibliotherapy were eventually given appointments, many reported that they no longer wanted treatment, as their symptoms had subsided. When they re-took Burns's mood inventories, they reported significantly less depression and anxiety than the group that did not receive his book while waiting. Furthermore, some of his research showed that the bibliotherapy groups reported as much improvement in mood and alleviation of symptoms as a therapy-only group that did not receive bibliotherapy.

Such "hands-on" books, offering step-by-step activities and exercises for therapists and clients alike, brought CBT into the self-help mainstream. During the last half-century, CBT titles have begun to populate the self-help shelves at bookstores, making CBT widely accepted as a model for self-help practices that millions can apply to their own lives even without engaging in therapy.

The Third Wave

Despite the popularity of CBT and the well-researched effectiveness of its methods in a wide variety of populations, some clients need still more tools to overcome treatment resistance. The third wave grew out of a difficulty in reaching some clients who lacked sufficient life skills and coping skills to deal with everyday life issues. Treatment-resistant populations with suicidal ideation, addictions, eating disorders, a history of abuse, or personality disorders needed something a bit more than CBT could offer. For these hard-to-reach populations, practices of CBT were combined with concepts originating in Eastern thought and spiritual practices, such as mindfulness, acceptance, emotional regulation, spirituality, dialectics, and practical skill building.

One of the most rapidly growing treatment modalities today for hard-to-reach clients, Dialectical Behavior Therapy, was developed by Marsha Linehan. DBT originated out of her work with severely impulsive suicidal patients. Realizing that many suicidal clients had characteristics of borderline personality disorder, she developed a treatment modality that combined the change-based skills of CBT with the acceptance-based skills of mindfulness. The word *dialectics* means opposites, underscoring the approach of DBT, which synthesizes and balances the opposite and conflicting emotions surrounding the need for change versus acceptance of the way things are. DBT offers a heavy psychoeducational treatment program filled with daily logs, diary cards, and daily practice of coping skills and strategies, which are often made easier with the help of various acronyms and mnemonics.

Other increasingly popular and well-researched third-wave treatment modalities are Acceptance and Commitment Therapy (ACT), developed by Steven Hayes, and Mindfulness-Based Cognitive Therapy (MBCT), the eight-week group-based treatment developed by Jon Kabat-Zinn, Philip Barnard, Zindel Segal, Mark Williams, and John Teasdale. All these relatively new approaches from the last quarter-century are unified in that they stress integrating CBT practices with mindfulness and acceptance strategies that focus on present-centered awareness. The chart below offers a summary of the major contributors and sample key concepts of the various approaches.

Figure I.1 The Three Waves of Psychological Treatment

Wave	Treatment Approach	Major Contributors	Sample of Key Concepts
First Wave	Behaviorism	B. F. Skinner Ivan Pavlov Joseph Wolpe	Reinforcement Token Economy Conditioning Behavioral Charts Systematic Desensitization Exposure Technique Relapse Prevention Stimulus Response
Second Wave	Rational Emotive Behavior Therapy Cognitive Behavior Therapy (CBT)	Albert Ellis Aaron Beck Judith Beck David Burns Matthew McKay Robert Leahy	Rational vs. Irrational Thinking Cognitive Distortions Coping Cards Core Irrational Beliefs Cognitive Restructuring Mood Logs Journals Worksheets Skills Practice
Third Wave	Dialectical Behavior Therapy (DBT) Acceptance and Commitment Therapy (ACT) Mindfulness-Based Cognitive Therapy (MBCT)	Marsha Linehan Stephen Hayes Matthew McKay Jon Kabat-Zinn	Acceptance Mindfulness Relaxation Distress Tolerance Interpersonal Effectiveness Present-Centered Awareness Cognitive Defusions Acronyms and Metaphors Diary Cards Worksheets Skills Practice

How This Book Is Organized

This book is designed to be user-friendly for you as the therapist, just as the solutions in this book are designed to be user-friendly for your clients. Each chapter has the same format to make it easy to look up a particular problem and find practical solutions for treatment. The structure is as follows:

Introduction. Each chapter introduction introduces one of the 10 most common client problems that provide the focus for this book.

Treatment Tips. This section provides a menu of tips and techniques to use with your clients based on current popular treatment trends, including CBT and third-wave approaches, specifically DBT, ACT, and MBCT.

A *Toolkit of Metaphors.* For each problem area, metaphorical objects represent solutions that you can share with your clients. Having clients use metaphorical objects to remind them of important therapeutic points offers a very effective practice for helping them alter habits of thinking and behavior. I use household and office items that can be purchased inexpensively (such as rubber bands to represent stress or Band-Aids to represent healing), as well as dollar-store or online novelty items that help me emphasize important psychological concepts. For example, for clients who tend to get angry and speak before they think things through, I provide a miniature stop sign that serves to remind them to stop and think before reacting. I urge them to stop and wait as they ask themselves, "What am I thinking?" or "What are the irrational thoughts?" For clients who find themselves all too often in conflict with spouses, children, or others close to them, I demonstrate a finger trap toy to remind them that trying to prove that they are "right" will get them stuck in the "trap." The couples I see have a lot of fun with this item and use this visual with one another as a reminder not to get caught in the trap of arguing.

Using metaphorical items has been extremely helpful in both individual and group treatment, and I often have clients assemble a metaphorical toolkit of various reminders of important therapeutic lessons. In my office, I have a supply of various items to choose from when I want to emphasize certain psychological points. Many clients have reported that they keep the items or toolkits that they have assembled during treatment in various prominent places, such as on their kitchen counter, on their desk at work, or in the glove compartment in their car, to serve as a daily reminder. A few clients have even made decorative displays of the metaphorical items by arranging them in pretty bowls or showcasing them in a shadow box mounted on the wall. Clients have shown me pictures of how they have displayed their meta-phorical toolkit items, and some have reported they use this activity with their own children to help them assemble their own life-skills toolkit. Clients who are teachers have used this activity with their students when teaching them life skills such as anger and stress management.

Therapeutic Takeaways. A checklist of solution-oriented takeaways summarizes each chapter.

Handouts. At the end of each chapter are handouts to offer your clients as practice opportunities between sessions. They can also be used for in-session psychoeducation. (Note: All handouts in the book are available for download on my website by following this link: http://www.belmontwellness.com/ultimate-solution -handouts/.)

Recommended Resources. The last page of each chapter offers recommendations for relevant clinician books, self-help bibliotherapy resources for clients, treatment tools, and web links to resources relating to recommendations from the chapter.

Recommended Resources

Clinician Books

Cognitive Behavior Therapy: Basics and Beyond
  Judith S. Beck
86 TIPS (Treatment Ideas & Practical Strategies) for the Therapeutic Toolbox
  Judith A. Belmont
103 Group Activities and TIPS (Treatment Ideas & Practical Strategies)
  Judith A. Belmont
127 More Amazing Tips and Tools for the Therapeutic Toolbox
  Judith A. Belmont
Ten Days to Self Esteem: The Leader's Manual
  David D. Burns

ACT Made Simple: A Quick-Start Guide to ACT Basics and Beyond
   Russ Harris
Self-Help That Works: Resources to Improve Emotional Health and Strengthen Relationships
   John C. Norcross, Linda F. Campbell, John M. Grohol, John W. Santrock. Florin Selagea, and Robert Sommer
The CBT Toolbox: A Workbook for Clients and Clinicians
   Jeff Riggenbach
The Big Book of ACT Metaphors: A Practitioner's Guide to Experiential Exercises & Metaphors in Acceptance and Commitment Therapy
   Jill A. Stoddard and Niloofar Afari
DBT Made Simple: A Quick-Start Guide to Help Clients
   Sheri Van Dijk

Links

Association for Contextual Behavioral Science
"Acceptance & Commitment Therapy (ACT)"
   http://contextualscience.org/act
Beck Institute for Cognitive Behavior Therapy
   http://www.beckinstitute.org
Belmont Wellness: Emotional Wellness for Positive Living
   http://www.belmontwellness.com/for-mental-health-professionals/
   psychoeducational-handouts-quizzes-group-activities/
The Linehan Institute: Behavioral Tech
(Dialectical Behavior Therapy)
   http://behavioraltech.org
Mindfulness-Based Cognitive Therapy
   http://mbct.com

CHAPTER ONE

The Stress Solution
Tension as Motivation

What do getting married, having a child, going on vacation, joining a competitive sports team, coming home for the holidays, applying to grad school, traveling, finding a new job, starting your own business, planning a celebration, and even just getting ready for a party all have in common?

All of these events—no matter how small or monumental they may seem—are examples of stress. Although stress typically carries a negative connotation, few of our clients want to avoid these stresses; in fact, many of them yearn to be stressed like that! Yet, all too often, stress is regarded as an undesirable menace to our mental and physical health. According to a study done by the American Psychological Association's American Institute of Stress (2013), 77% of people surveyed regularly experienced physical symptoms caused by stress, 73% admitted to psychological symptoms caused by stress, and 48% believed that stress had a negative impact on their lives. In studies like these, it is assumed that stress is negatively affecting us, rather than propelling us to lead a happier and more vibrant life.

Whether our clients seek counseling for depression, anxiety, or relationship problems, the topic of stress is very much intertwined with their issues, and how to manage their stress becomes a common focus of treatment. Consider the case of Natalie, a 34-year-old woman who came for counseling feeling depressed and experiencing very low self-esteem. Her stress was partly a result of her keeping her thoughts and feelings to herself while being a sounding board for others. She kept so much of her own pain, memories, and trauma from childhood inside that the stress she felt was distancing her from others and causing her to feel resentful toward those close to her, leading to more stress as the tension built. As she learned that the stress she was feeling could give her the motivation she needed to open up to those close to her about her feelings of loneliness and sadness, she started to let down her guard, and the more she was able to trust others, the more her negative stress level decreased. Her high level of suppression finally gave her the push she needed to ask for help rather than only to give it. At first she felt more vulnerable and less "safe," as she found it hard to trust others, but as she expressed herself more, she became less fearful of others' reactions and more focused on her goal of having the courage to express her feelings. She began to trust herself more, which in turn helped her to trust others. As she gave herself permission to show some "weakness" and share her thoughts and feelings, her relationships improved and she was able to be less self-critical. As her tension and stress lifted, so did her depression. She realized that it was a sign of courage to show that she was not always strong, and that the tension of keeping things in for so long was really a self-imposed exile that might have been adaptive in her abusive childhood but was no longer a positive survival skill.

This example shows the importance of helping clients learn how to use their stress to motivate themselves rather than to hold themselves back. Their tension becomes a warning and a motivator to create a better life. Therapists are in the unique position of being able to help clients embrace stress as actually desirable, and to view it as just a part of a full life. We can educate our clients that stress can actually be quite positive, something to be sought after rather than avoided.

One thing I have found useful for clients who claim they feel "stressed out" is the self-test in Handout 1.4 ("Where's Your Sense of Humor? Take a Humor Inventory").This short quiz helps to give clients the message that a sense of humor is an important ingredient in handling stress. It can be fun for your clients to fill the self-test out between sessions and then bring it in for you to review at the beginning of the next session. After all, part of the reason our clients get "stressed out" is that they lose their sense of humor and take life and themselves too seriously. This self-test underscores the important lesson that humor is a great stress reliever.

It's important not to forget the importance of modeling a sense of humor ourselves. In attempting to impart a sense of humor—as in teaching any other lesson—showing by example is our most effective tool. A therapeutic manner that incorporates a sense of humor goes a long way.

In the treatment tips section in this chapter, I offer some of the demonstrations and activities that I use to help clients embrace stress instead of trying to escape it. The activities in this section will help you help your clients see that, when we welcome just the right amount of tension and excitement in our lives, our lives can become more interesting and fulfilling.

As stress pioneer Hans Selye emphasized, stress just is. Although we often view stress as coming from the outside, much of our stress is a result of what goes on between our ears. Because stress is an inside job, educating your clients about it will give them more control over the stress in their lives.

This introduction to stress gives you a foundation for imparting knowledge to your client about the usefulness of stress in their lives. "Common Myths About Stress" (Handout 1.1) provides information about stress to you and your client. Another useful handout, "Tips for Managing Stress—Not Carrying It!" (Handout 1.3) helps educate clients about how they can more effectively manage stress.

In this chapter, as well as in others, a psychoeducational approach using demonstrations and metaphors can you help you make an impact with your client regarding important life lessons. It's one thing to inform your clients about facts and myths about stress; it's another thing to show them and involve them. Active involvement in activities helps make the learning come alive and teaches skills in a way that words alone can't do.

I have found that showing clients how stress can be positive is a real eye opener, and very helpful in encouraging them to look for and make use of the advantages of stress in their lives. Since most clients find stress challenging at best, knowledge about how stress can be positive comes as a welcome relief, particularly when clients are overwhelmed by work and life demands and see no end in sight. For instance, 42-year old Gail was a bundle of nerves when she came to my office. She told me she couldn't take the stress any longer, and she was physically getting sick. The stress of her work life was compounded by the problems she was experiencing with her teenager at home as well as lingering custody issues with her ex-husband. The effects on her body were multiple. She found herself overeating to the point of becoming mildly obese. As she began to feel increasingly uncomfortable with her weight, she developed the attitude that there was no point in exercising. She would tell herself, *"What's the use? I'll always be this way and things will never get better."*

In addition to overeating, she had a habit of depending on wine with dinner to "relax." Food and wine were all too comforting to her, and in times of stress she reached for more, which of course made her feel worse about herself, since she gained more and more weight. With the extra weight, she felt lethargic and depressed in addition to her feelings of stress.

Her shame about her behavior prevented her from being truthful with her friends and family, and she went so far as to suggest to them that her weight gain was the result of a thyroid problem and early meno-pause. She wouldn't ask for help because she felt "pathetic" and "weak." She finally decided to get some counseling, although she felt quite hope-less that there was anything anybody could do to make her life less stressful.

I used various techniques with Gail to help her figure out strategies for reacting to her stress more positively, instead of reaching for food and wine. I helped her to challenge her "all-or-nothing" perspective that exercise would not help, and she started to make small steps toward beginning a regular exercise plan that could fit into her hectic life. I used handouts such as "Examples of Depression and Anxiety-Producing Cognitive Distortions" (Handout 2.3, in Chapter 2) to help her identify her pattern of thinking errors. Sheets like these helped her to uncover her own cognitive distor-tions, or thinking errors, such as her erroneous use of "fortune telling" ("I'll always be this way and things will never get better") and "labeling" (describ-ing herself as "pathetic" and "weak.") Since I find that bibliotherapy is extremely important in offering structure between sessions, I recommended Geneen Roth's *When Food Is Love* (1991) to help Gail uncover some of the psychological issues underlying her emotional eating, as well as Judith Beck's *The Beck Diet Solution* (2008), which applies practical cognitive behavior therapy (CBT) self-help strategies to weight loss. I encouraged her to break through her isolation and reconnect with friends and be more open to making new ones. Part of her psychoeducation was to learn that stress could motivate her, not just debilitate her, and to learn how to make stress work for her rather than against her. I encouraged her to learn to make stress her friend so that she could grow and heal as a person.

The next step with Gail was to do the "Weighing Pluses and Minuses" activity, which is further spelled out in the treatment tips section. In this exercise, I list with my clients the different ways they describe stress, and then they put minus and positive signs next to each item. They see that stress can be both positive and negative, and the activity disputes the myth that stress is mostly bad or negative. The "Weighing Pluses and Minuses" activity helps clients to identify their unique view of stress, including their misunderstandings, and to develop insight into how to see their stress in more positive ways. They learn that stress largely results from their perceptions about outside events, not the events themselves.

Treatment Tips

Now that your clients have learned how sweet stress can be, and appreciate how it can be a positive motivator, here are some mini-lessons, demonstrations, and activities to further help them embrace stress in their lives. I find that short lessons are very important in effective treatment, as our clients are not armed with the knowledge that we have, and knowledge becomes power. I like to back up my mini-lessons with a handout or worksheet, reinforcing their learning with at-home learning opportunities. Armed with many tools for stress management, such as the ones in this section, our clients find ways to thrive under stress—not just to survive.

☑ Activity: Weighing Pluses and Minuses

Have your clients write down at least 10 responses to the following phrase:

Stress is _____ .

Common responses include:

Stress is:

> *exhausting*
>
> *frustrating*
>
> *tiring*
>
> *too much to do*
>
> *difficult*
>
> *money problems*
>
> *coworkers*
>
> *customers*
>
> *kids*
>
> *in-laws*

Now instruct your clients to put a plus sign (+) or a minus sign (−) next to each item to convey whether they regard the answer as positive or negative. Let them know that some items are a mixed bag and can be both plus and minus. (In a group setting, you can make the list on a flip chart or board.)

The impact of seeing mostly minuses drives home the point that people often regard stress as negative, which in turn creates more stress. Point out that even items such as *too much to do* can be seen as positive because the absence of having things to do means depression and despondency, in which you are not challenged and involved. If there is a minus next to "in-laws," remember that the only reason people have in-laws is that they are married. Doesn't that deserve a positive? Likewise, you might remind clients who include customers and coworkers on the list as a source of negative stress, that they can also be considered positive—without them, there would be no job! And as for stress over kids—which is often regarded as negative—parents generally would agree that the joys of having their children outweigh the day-to-day stresses and hassles.

This simple yet effective exercise helps clients to embrace the stress in their lives. In this way, they can be encouraged to be more objective and positive about stress and to see stress as a motivator in their lives and as a key to success rather than a hindrance to it.

☑ *Activity: Traits of Stress Managers and Stress Carriers*
Another useful activity to do with your client is to follow up "Weighing Pluses and Minuses" with brainstorming a listing of the traits of a *stress manager* and a *stress carrier*. The difference? People who handle stress well manage their stress. People who don't manage their stress well tend to spend more time giving it to everyone else! Ironically, these are generally the people who think that they have no stress! If you type this list on a tablet or laptop, you can send it to your client to use as a handout that you made together. Or, using the list below as a template, you can make your own list as a handout for clients.

Here are some ideas to include:

Stress Managers:	Stress Carriers:
Believe stress is positive	Believe stress is negative
Embrace stress	Try to avoid stress
Make self-care a priority	Are too busy to attend to self-care
Set limits on their time and energy	Do too much, then feel exhausted
Value and nurture relationships	Neglect connecting with others
Have patience	Are rushed
Are calm and confident	Feel anxious and pressured
Control and manage their time	Are controlled by time (there's ever enough of it!)

☑ *Mini-Lesson: Kobasa's 3 Cs of the Stress-Hardy Personality*
Educating your clients about the 3 Cs of hardiness can help them make stress their friend. The 3 Cs are based on the work of Suzanne Kobasa (1979), who did research on the stress-hardy personality. In her studies of executives and those with stressful occupations, she found that those who were healthiest both psychologically and physically exhibited the characteristics she referred to as the "3 Cs":

Commitment. Those who feel a sense of commitment have a feeling of involvement in something outside themselves. Therefore, they tend not to feel isolated but rather to sense that their actions have a purpose and contribute to the greater good.

Control. This is perhaps the key factor in emotional health—a sense that you can control the things you can, without trying to control others. Rather than feeling like a victim of circumstances or a pawn in the lives of others, stress-hardy people feel an internal locus of control.

Challenge. In the face of adversity, stress-resilient people typically feel challenged instead of overwhelmed. They are growth oriented and eager to meet new challenges.

I have used this concept many times with clients who have felt overwhelmed by stress. "The 3 Cs of Stress Hardiness" (Handout 1.2) at the end of this chapter will give your clients an opportunity to improve their own stress hardiness based on Kobasa's 3 Cs. The 3 Cs provide an easy way for them to remember the importance of focusing on what is under their control in life, to see how they can grow through life's challenges, and to recognize the importance of committing themselves to pursuits in life that they believe in and that give them a sense of contributing to the world.

☑ Mini-Lesson: Making Peace with Life's Dialectics

I enjoy using treatment practices from various models of treatment, and Dialectical Behavior Therapy (DBT) gives me many practical treatment tools to put in my therapeutic toolbox. DBT and other third-wave therapies offer perspectives that CBT does not. This rapidly growing treatment modality is based on the idea that we all experience conflicts in everyday life in response to our opposing needs, wants, feelings, thoughts, and behaviors. The term *dialectics* means "opposites," and the heavily psychoeducational DBT approach provides strategies to help clients make peace with the dialectics in their lives.

DBT's name is an example of a dialectic. This popular form of psychotherapy is an outgrowth of seemingly opposite treatment orientations, uniting the traditionally Western approach of Cognitive Behavior Therapy with the Eastern practices of mindfulness and meditation. In DBT, West meets East as Skinner and Beck meet Buddha, combining the dialectal conflict of the need to change with the need to accept things as they are.

As we help our clients understand the dialectics of life and the contradictions and conflicting emotions that are inevitably part of life, they learn to regard opposing feelings and thoughts as normal. An awareness of life's dialectics will help lessen stress by allowing clients to let go of the expectation that life should be free of conflict and welcome the realization that life is full of tension, both positive and negative. This fundamental understanding helps clients embrace conflicts in their lives and manage their stress instead of carrying it.

"Making Peace With the Dialectics of Life" (Handout 1.5) and "Life's Dialectics in the Form of Oxymorons" (Handout 1.6) are handout supplements designed to help clients grasp these points. These sheets offer opportunities to have fun with the concept of dialectics. I have used these types of mini-lessons and handouts frequently with clients, as they emphasize the importance of creative and flexible thinking skills. Worksheets such as these normalize the dialectics in everyday life and help clients make peace with their conflicting emotions and needs.

☑ Visualization: Using Metaphors to Effectively Cope with Stress

Using metaphors to represent life's paradoxes can further help clients manage their stress. Metaphors use imagery to help unlock emotions, and using imagery can help people picture concepts in a way that words can't convey. Use of metaphors is a vital part of a solution-oriented therapeutic approach. With some flexible thinking and creativity, it's not hard to find metaphors to illustrate lessons.

As coauthor of *The Swiss Cheese Theory of Life* (Belmont & Shor, 2012), I enjoy giving demonstrations where I use a wedge of Swiss cheese to illustrate the unpredictability of life. In working with individuals, even if it's not practical to bring in a wedge of cheese, I have the client visualize Swiss cheese to make the point that life isn't supposed to be so smooth and predictable like cream cheese or American. Rather, life is full of holes, and likewise, life is full of challenges to get through. I emphasize that the larger the holes in the Swiss, the more flavorful and stronger the cheese. Likewise, the bigger the holes in our lives, the bigger our challenges and the more we can develop our character and uniqueness, as long as we "deepen and don't weaken."

I also use finger-trap carnival toys, purchased from an online novelty distributor, to demonstrate various points, such as how people get stuck in traps when they argue and try to prove they are right. This is a great metaphor and visualization for an argumentative couple. I sometimes give my clients a metaphorical prop to bring home to remind them of the lesson. ACT founder Stephen Hayes uses the finger trap to demonstrate how people get stuck if they refuse to accept some degree of unavoidable pain in their lives. The more they resist what is, the more they get stuck by refusing to accept things beyond their control.

One of my favorite demonstrations regarding stress uses a rubber band, and I always have rubber bands on hand in my desk so I can show this lesson to clients. (You can also use a balloon to demonstrate the same thing.) I show them that when the rubber band is not stretched at all, it is limp and does not have a useful function. However, too much stretch can cause the band to snap. The happy medium lies somewhere in between, where the band has some stretch and "give" without being too limp or too stretched. This represents the balance that we seek in our lives in terms of stress. We want some stress to spice up our lives, but not so much that we become overwhelmed and "snap." I give my clients rubber bands to take home to help them keep in mind that stress is good in moderation.

I use the visualization of a stringed instrument to further make my point. If the string on a guitar, for example, is not tightened enough, the music will drone. However, if the string is wound too tightly, the pitch will be too high, or the string might even snap. It is only with the right amount of tension on the string that we can play beautiful music.

Quick visualizations that make a therapeutic point are more effective than words alone. When clients visualize something—and even better, when they experience it—it produces more of an impact and they are more likely to remember the concept being taught. The "Toolkit of Metaphors for Treating Stress" at the end of the chapter offers other metaphors to represent how to deal with stress.

☑ Activity: Stress Resiliency Through Acceptance and Mindfulness Practice

A discussion on stress without mentioning the important of relaxation and mindfulness techniques would make this chapter incomplete. In the last few decades, mindfulness exercises have been a staple in virtually all third-wave cognitive behavioral treatment approaches. Mindfulness practice is a vital key to stress reduction. Mindfulness practices include some type of relaxation training or practice to cope with negative stress for emotional and physical health. Acceptance and Commitment Therapy (ACT), DBT, and Mindfulness-Based Cognitive Therapy (MBCT) are all anchored in the foundation of mindfulness practice. Bringing mindfulness techniques into stress-reduction practices became mainstream when cardiologist Dr. Herbert Benson outlined a meditative technique called the "Relaxation Response" (Benson, 1975). His medical approach to meditation and his focus on the physiological benefits of relaxation practice accepted by the Western medical community demystified the practice and distilled it enough that it could be accessible to the mainstream population. As founder of the Benson-Henry Institute for Mind Body Medicine at Massachusetts General Hospital in Boston, Benson is responsible for integrating Eastern spiritual meditative practices into modern-day medicine. Benson focused on meditative techniques to decrease stress and improve health to ward off heart disease and other health stress-related disorders, such as gastrointestinal ailments, insomnia, and hypertension. Benson's premise was that meditative techniques release chemicals and brain signals to reduce tension. In his hallmark book, *The Relaxation Response*, Benson outlined the major ingredients to stress reduction through relaxation training to quiet the mind and body.

The major elements of relaxation practice are as follows:

1. Find a quiet place that can be visited on a regular basis, and once or twice daily sit comfortably for 10 to 20 minutes.
2. Closing your eyes, focus on one word, such as *one*. Repeat this word over and over.
3. Progressively relax the body, either by focusing on various parts of the body and intentionally relaxing them or by tightening and then releasing the muscles.
4. Strive to maintain a non-judgmental, passive attitude as you observe sensations, not judge them. Let thoughts come and go.

Benson paved the way for third-wave treatments to be embraced by modern medicine and psychological practice. Some practitioners who are trained in and comfortable with teaching mindfulness guide their clients with mindfulness and relaxation exercises in session. I personally use such exercises in group settings, and in individual settings refer my clients to the books and CDs included in the "Recommended Resources" section, which offer many self-help variations of relaxation and mindfulness practice. One of the more widely used is the *Guided Mindfulness Meditation* three-part CD series by MBCT founder Jon Kabat-Zinn.

☑ Activity: Skill-Building Logs and Handouts
for Stress Resiliency

Worksheets and daily or weekly stress logs offer your clients opportunities to practice managing stress and give them structured opportunities to track their progress. As emphasized before, most psychoeducational approaches—such as CBT, DBT, ACT, and MCBT—emphasize the importance of between-session homework. Filling out diaries, logs, and worksheets is vital to any type of solution-oriented therapy. The important thing to note is that, just as when learning a new language or learning to ride a bike or drive a car, you won't really be able to learn to manage stress without practice. The solution-oriented therapist needs to offer these tools so that clients can practice skills between sessions. "Stress Log" and "Completed Stress Log Sample" (Handouts 1.7 and 1.8) and "Stress Journal" (Handout 1.9) provide opportunities for between-session practice that can be reviewed during following sessions.

☑ *Activity: Assembling a Stress Toolkit*

This is my most popular activity regarding stress. When conducting group sessions, I bring in a variety of objects for assembling a stress kit, with each object serving as a metaphor for some aspect of stress. I purchase these inexpensive objects at places like the supermarket, the drugstore, the dollar store, or a discount online novelty store. I offer my clients small plastic bags that they can fill with various items to take home to remind them of the lessons they learned in the group.

I also keep many metaphorical objects in my office to illustrate various points. These metaphoric visualizations have been very helpful therapeutically, and I use them often.

A Toolkit of Metaphors for Treating Stress

The following are ideas of what goes in the Stress Management Toolkit:

Small rubber Super Ball. The harder it is thrown on the ground, the higher it bounces. Stress-resilient people don't focus on how hard they fall, but on how hard and how high they bounce back.

Rubber band. If the band is pulled too much, it will snap. If it is pulled too little, it remains limp and nonfunctional. Just the right amount of tension allows the band to be functional without snapping.

Slinky. It goes in all different directions and is very adaptable and flexible.

Paintbrush. Your attitude is your mind's paintbrush—it colors your world.

Candy kiss. Be good to others and give others a kiss! Good connections with others will help you be more stress-resilient.

Cartoon clip. Having a sense of humor helps in warding off negative stress.

Stress ball. Stress balls teach us a lot about the stress-hardy personality. They roll with the punches, retain their shape even when squeezed, have no rough edges, stay afloat, and are soft and flexible.

Can you and your clients add to this toolkit?

Therapeutic Takeaways

☑ Teach your clients that stress is neither good nor bad—it just "is." Our perceptions determine what *stresses us out*.

☑ Help your clients realize the importance of a sense of humor in stress relief.

☑ Use short activities such as "Weighing Pluses and Minuses" to educate clients about stress and help them to process what they have learned.

☑ Teach your clients that life is full of conflicting opposites— or dialectics—that cause tension that needs to be embraced rather than avoided. This is the basic premise underlying Dialectical Behavior Therapy.

☑ Mindfulness is an acceptance-based practice that is used for stress management training with clients. It is characterized by non-judgmental and present-focused awareness.

☑ Use metaphors liberally with clients to demonstrate psychological lessons, and keep metaphorical objects handy for demonstrations in treatment.

Handouts

The following worksheets will help your clients build their stress-resiliency skills. These handouts are all related to the lessons of this chapter. As a general guideline, handouts and assignments are given to clients at the end of the session as homework, unless they are used in the session itself to illustrate points. Make sure you leave ample time to go over your expectations regarding use of the selected handouts.

When you give out assignments, it is important to follow up with your clients at the beginning of the next session to review and discuss their homework. Going over the homework is an essential aspect of being a solution-oriented therapist.

Note: All handouts in the book are available for download on my website by following the link below: http://www.belmontwellness.com/ultimate-solution-handouts/

Handout 1.1: Common Myths About Stress

Myth 1: Most stress is caused outside of ourselves.

Do people stress you out? Does traffic stress you out? Does snow stress you out?

Usually, people will answer yes to these questions. Yet, in actuality, stress comes from within ourselves—not from the outside.

The truth is that no one has the power to make you stressed unless you give it to them. Traffic is just traffic. If you were a traffic control officer, that would be your livelihood—no traffic, no job. Likewise, if you were a ski instructor or lift operator, no snow would mean no work. Talk about stress!

Myth 2: Stress is not controllable—it controls us.

Our stress is largely a result of our interpretations. By controlling our perceptions, we control our stress.

Still not sure? Consider the following example.

Imagine that you're taking a shower and the water is lukewarm. Many of us would feel very stressed and experience a range of emotions on a continuum from annoyance to outright anger. It could prove to be a stressful start to what would otherwise be an uneventful day. Now, consider the same shower with the same water temperature. However, this time you know that the hot water heater is broken and expect that the water will be cold until the repairman comes later in the day. The same lukewarm water, expected to be cold, is a positive surprise rather than a source of annoyance. Thus, the negative stress is replaced by a sense of relief, and you enjoy your shower with a sense of gratitude.

Myth 3: Most people find the same things stressful.

Stress is not the same for everyone—and the greater the degree of baseline resiliency a person possesses, the more he or she will find stress motivating rather than debilitating. Consider the adage "One's man's meat is another man's poison." What is stressful for one person is invigorating for another. Whereas some of us find the idea of skydiving, ziplining, or skiing on an expert trail terrifying, a more adventurous soul will be exhilarated by the stress. Some people seek to repeat the very same experiences that many of us would avoid at all costs.

Myth 4: Stress is bad for you.

Despite the common misperception, stress is not bad for you. To quote Hans Selye, the pioneer of the study of stress, "Stress is the spice of life." We need stress to feel engaged. In fact, trying to escape or avoid stress will make life more stressful!

Selye differentiated between negative and positive stress: He actually referred to positive stress as "Eustress" and referred to negative stress as "Distress." Thus, stress is not good or bad—it just *is*. It is our perceptions that make it seem bad! According to Selye, "Adopting the right attitude can convert a negative stress into a positive one."

Myth 5: Stress interferes with success.

Negative stress can be debilitating, but stress itself is not inherently bad. It's stress that is not properly managed that leads to impairment, illness, and even death. Positive stress, however, can be exhilarating and motivating. From youth soccer to the NFL—and everywhere in between—stress motivates players to win. Would people buy high-priced tickets to watch their favorite major league sports team play if they already knew the outcome of the game? Would we really want to know the score ahead of time? What makes watching a game exciting and thrilling is the stress of the unknown.

Myth 6: Stress is hazardous to your health.

Stress, in itself, is not necessarily hazardous. It's how you adapt to stress that determines whether it affects your mind and body. For example, for the Type A stress-ridden personality, there is a correlation between being hard driving and experiencing heart disease, high blood pressure, and even early death. In contrast, the Type B personality is considered to be more relaxed and low-key, and was once thought to be associated with a longer life. However, later studies have shown that it is really the hostility factor that determines whether stress is actually detrimental to our health. Unbridled hostility and anger have been found to be the factors that determine whether stress motivates you or breaks you down. Your anger level is really the determinant—not the stress itself.

Handout 1.2: The 3 Cs of Stress Hardiness
Based on the work of Suzanne Kobasa (1979)

Commitment. Those who feel a sense of commitment have a sense of involvement in something outside themselves. They are committed to a purpose and a greater good and are working toward something they believe in.

Control. This is perhaps the key factor in emotional health—a sense that you can control the things you can. *However, that does not mean controlling others!* Rather than feeling a victim of circumstance, stress-hardy people feel in control of their lives.

Challenge. In the face of adversity, people feel challenged instead of overwhelmed. They are growth oriented and eager to meet new challenges.

The following questions will help you to personalize and process these 3 Cs.

Ways I can feel more involved and committed:

_____

_____

Ways I can feel more "in control":

_____

_____

Ways I can feel more challenged:

_____

_____

Handout 1.3: Tips for Managing Stress—Not Carrying It!

Change your perceptions, change your life.

The biggest stressor comes not from the outside, but from between our ears. There are some things we can't change, but we can change our perceptions! Shift your focus to what can be changed, not to what can't be changed. Our thoughts create our stress. Over 80% of our life is determined not by events, but by our reactions to them. Remember to stick to the facts, not interpretations. Often we can't "get over" something because of stories we tell ourselves.

Make an effort to think more positively.

Remind yourself that stress can be positive. If we put a negative spin on it, then it will be negative. It has been estimated that the average person thinks well-over 50,000 thoughts per day. If even 10% are negative thoughts, which is an underestimate for most people, that comes to 5,000 negative thoughts a day! Start the day with the intention to think positively about your stress.

Don't forget the importance of humor!

When we feel under stress, a sense of humor is often one of the first things to go. Smiling, laughing, and looking at the light side of life can do wonders for our mental health. Look on the light side of life at every opportunity.

Take care of yourself mentally and physically.

Practice self-care techniques and attempt to nurture and nourish your body as well as your mind. Eating well and exercising will help you keep your stress under control and you will feel healthier in mind and body.

Don't be too hard on yourself—or on others either.

People who truly like themselves and look for the good in others are far less stressed than people who are judgmental. Accept imperfections, mistakes, and even failures in yourself and others with kindness and compassion. Compassion goes a long way toward soothing the mind and soul.

Focus on what is in your control, not what is beyond it.

Think of the Serenity Prayer by Reinhold Niebuhr: "God grant me the serenity to accept the things I cannot change; the courage to change the things I can; and the wisdom to know the difference." Those who focus on what is in their control are more stress-hardy and more likely to grow from stress.

Challenge and commit yourself to do what you love.

People who are energized by pursuits they love and to which they are committed are generally more stress-hardy. Finding meaning in your daily life, in paid or unpaid work, working toward making the world a better place, and finding a passion that you can contribute to the world all lead to stress hardiness.

Connect with others—don't isolate!

Establishing warm and supportive relationships with people, family, friends, coworkers, and neighbors can reduce negative stress immensely. Self-disclosure helps to manage stress rather than let it build up.

Handout 1.4: Where's Your Sense of Humor?
Take a Humor Inventory

The following questions will help you take stock of your "humor inventory."

Rate each item on the following scale of 1 to 5:

False_____True
| 1 | 2 | 3 | 4 | 5 |

_____ 1. I take myself too seriously.

_____ 2. I am too busy to find the humor in things.

_____ 3. I am too involved with "important things" to be able to see the lighter side of life.

_____ 4. I am worried about what others think about me.

_____ 5. On average, I do not laugh a lot.

_____ 6. There is not much that strikes me as funny.

_____ 7. I have not had a good laugh in quite some time.

Take your total score and divide it by 7:

Total score _____ divided by 7 equals your score: _____ .

Interpretation of Your Score

1 Superb: Your Humor Quotient is unusually high! Keep up the good work!
2 Very Good: You have a very good ability to see the lightness in life!
3 Average: Your Humor Quotient could use some boosting.
4 Needs Work: Look for more opportunities to lighten your load.
5 Needs a *Lot* of Work: Life is too serious to be taken so seriously! Try to find more lightness in your life! If your mood is low, consider getting professional help.

What are some ways that you can improve your Humor Quotient?

Handout 1.5: Making Peace With the Dialectics of Life

Life is full of "dialectics," which means that life is fraught with constant stress and tension due to conflicting wants, needs, emotions, behaviors, and thoughts. Stress is a by-product of those conflicts between opposing needs and wants. Learning to accept and embrace conflicting emotions and thoughts will increase inner peace of mind.

These are some of life's dialectics that are familiar to many of us:

- The more love you give, the more love you often receive.
- The most controlling people are the most out of control.
- The more we cling to someone, the more we push him or her away.
- The more we seek happiness, the more it eludes our grasp.
- Sometimes we need to lose ourselves to find ourselves.
- Often, the more we feel isolated, the more we avoid intimacy for fear of rejection.
- The more you accept that life is difficult, the less difficult it will be.
- You want to eat healthier, but you can't resist the drive-in window.

Now it's your turn—fill in your own dialectics.

_____

_____

_____

_____

_____

Handout 1.6: Life's Dialectics in the Form of Oxymorons

Life is full of paradoxes—that's what makes it so interesting!

Even in our everyday life we use terms called *oxymorons*—dialectical, paradoxical phrases. They are so commonly accepted that we don't usually realize that they contain two opposites!

Jumbo shrimp
Filthy rich
Bittersweet
Lovesick
Definite maybe
Living dead
Little while
Guest host
Deafening silence

Can you think of more?

_____
_____
_____
_____

Handout 1.7: Stress Log

This Stressful Event Log will help you analyze, understand, and manage your stress more effectively. Keep a stress log regularly to help yourself manage your stress . . . *and not carry it!*

Using the completed form in Handout 1.8 as a sample, fill in the spaces below using a stressful situation from your life.

Stressful Event Description	
Negative Emotions	Positive Emotions
Strength of Negative Emotions 1 2 3 4 5 6 7 8 9 10 Low　　　　　　　　High	Strength of Positive Emotions 1 2 3 4 5 6 7 8 9 10 Low　　　　　　　　High
Identify Negative Beliefs	Challenge With Positive Beliefs
Type of Cognitive Distortion	Healthy Alternative
Certainty of Your Beliefs 1 2 3 4 5 6 7 8 9 10 Low　　　　　　　　High	Certainty of Your Beliefs 1 2 3 4 5 6 7 8 9 10 Low　　　　　　　　High
Unhealthy Behaviors	Healthy Behaviors
Cost/Benefit Analysis: Unhealthy Coping	Cost/Benefit Analysis: Healthy Coping
My Conclusions and Goals	

Handout 1.8: Completed Stress Log Sample

Stressful Event Description Making a presentation for a meeting at work	
Negative Emotions Anxiety, fear	**Positive Emotions** Excited for the opportunity, energized
Strength of Negative Emotions _____X_____ 1 2 3 4 5 6 7 8 9 10 Low High	**Strength of Positive Emotions** _____X_____ 1 2 3 4 5 6 7 8 9 10 Low High
Identify Negative Beliefs They might not agree with me. It would be awful if I got tongue-tied! I wish I was as smart as Nancy.	**Challenge With Positive Beliefs** Even if they don't, it wouldn't be terrible. It would be frustrating, but not a tragedy. Nancy's intelligence doesn't diminish my own; we are different.
Type of Cognitive Distortion Catastrophizing; comparisons	**Healthy Alternative** Sticking to the facts, not interpretations
Certainty of Your Beliefs _____X_____ 1 2 3 4 5 6 7 8 9 10 Low High	**Certainty of Your Beliefs** _____X____ 1 2 3 4 5 6 7 8 9 10 Low High
Unhealthy Behaviors Withdrawing before meetings Getting snippy with the family	**Healthy Behaviors** Practicing in front of a mirror Outlining my main points on a note card
Cost/Benefit Analysis: Unhealthy Coping Costs: Alienates others; causes conflict. Benefits: Keeps people away; protects me.	**Cost/Benefit Analysis: Healthy Coping** Costs: Takes time to plan. Benefits: Helps me feel empowered, organized, and prepared. Boosts my confidence.
My Conclusions and Goals By challenging my irrational beliefs and replacing them with more rational thoughts, I will use this presentation as an opportunity to grow healthier.	

Handout 1.9: Stress Journal

Date(s): _____

1. Stressful event(s)

_____

2. Emotional responses

_____

3. Degree of negative stress   LOW 1 2 3 4 5 6 7 8 9 10 HIGH

4. Degree of positive stress   LOW 1 2 3 4 5 6 7 8 9 10 HIGH

5. Unhealthy and healthy thoughts

_____

6. Unhealthy and healthy reactions

_____

7. What have I learned from my stress logs?

_____

8. Relaxation and mindfulness skills I have practiced

_____

9. Metaphors and visualizations I have used

_____

10. Examples of both positive and negative stress

_____

Recommended Resources

CDs

Goodbye Worries: Train Your Mind to Quiet Your Thoughts Anytime
Calming Collection, with Roberta Shapiro

Guided Mindfulness Meditation: Series 1 , Series 2 and Series 3
Jon Kabat-Zinn

Progressive Relaxation and Breathing
Matthew McKay and Patrick Fanning

Progressive Muscle Relaxation: 20 Minutes to Total Relaxation
Beth Salcedo

Self-Help Books

Stress without Distress
Hans Selye

The Relaxation Response
Herbert Benson

The Relaxation & Stress Reduction Workbook
Martha Davis, Elizabeth Robbins Eshelman, and Matthew McKay

The Stress and Relaxation Handbook: A Practical Guide to Self-Help Techniques
Jane Madders

A Mindfulness-Based Stress Reduction Workbook
Bob Stahl and Elisha Goldstein

Useful Links

About.com
"Stress Management"
stress.about.com

American Institute of Stress
http://www.stress.org

Change Your Thoughts, Change Your Life (blog)
http://www.stevenaitchison.co.uk/blog/

Mind Tools
"Stress Management Techniques"
http://www.mindtools.com/pages/main/newMN_TCS.htm

Psych Central

"Stress Management: Coping With Stress" by John H. Grohol
    http://psychcentral.com/stress/

Statistic Brain

"Stress Statistics"
    http://www.statisticbrain.com/stress-statistics/

CHAPTER TWO

The Anxiety Solution
Calming Irrational Fears

Considering that anxiety disorders affect 18% of the population (40 million adults) in America (Anxiety and Depression Association of America, n.d.), it is not surprising that anxiety is the reason that many of our clients seek counseling. Substance abuse, depression, and many other disorders are rooted, as well as manifested, in symptoms of anxiety. Our propensity for anxiety is due partly to our biological wiring and partly to environmental factors, such as being raised in an anxious household or a home with perfectionistic standards.

Regardless of biological and environmental predisposition, there is no shortage of opportunities in life for worry, and the variations of worrying are endless. Any gamut of events threatening your mental stability, safety, and happiness, and that of those close to you, is fodder for worry. Whether it is realistic or unrealistic worry, it takes a toll. Some real-life worry constitutes a response to problems that need to be solved, while many other types of worry fall in the *what if* category. Anxiety is more of this type, focusing on life's *could be* and *should be* possibilities, endless mental churning leads to little resolution or inner peace.

Some of the most common anxiety disorders that we see as clinicians are generalized anxiety disorder (GAD), posttraumatic stress disorder (PTSD), panic, specific phobias, and social anxiety disorder (SAD). According to the Anxiety and Depression Association of America, specific phobias are the most prevalent, affecting 19 million Americans

(8.7% of the population). Despite there being such a high prevalence of these phobias, specific phobias do not generally prompt individuals to seek professional help, since people who have fears of snakes, heights, or other specific stimuli generally take precautions to avoid exposure in everyday life. The time we see clients with specific phobias is when the phobia involves something our clients can't avoid, such as driving over bridges or in tunnels, or using elevators in the case of a client who lives or works on a building's upper floor which makes taking the stairs impractical.

Often, phobias and panic disorder are outgrowths of the very common generalized anxiety disorder (GAD), affecting 6.8 adults in America (3.1% of the population; Anxiety and Depression Association of America, n.d.). GAD is characterized by exaggerated, persistent, and unrealistic worry, and is a common reason that people seek help. Perhaps the most common type of anxiety disorder we see as clinicians is Social Anxiety Disorder (SAD). This is a form of extreme self-consciousness and overwhelming shyness in which those affected are painfully afraid of being judged or criticized. Also called social phobia, this disorder causes people to have trouble making friends and getting close to people. Their fear of embarrassing themselves interferes with their everyday functioning on the job and in their personal lives. The effects of SAD are crippling to our clients, and it is not uncommon for anxiety to be manifested in substance abuse as an attempt to self-medicate.

For example, John was a man in his late 60s who came to counseling when cardiac issues prompted him to give up alcohol after 40 years of daily use. Having just retired as a successful businessman, he found that even the simplest activities, such as going out to lunch with his wife, caused excessive anxiety. He felt as if all eyes were on him, and he was afraid of being criticized or judged. Although he had been quite sociable in the past, he now found social situations terrifying, and he felt he could hardly speak when in a group situation with unfamiliar people. Without alcohol as a social lubricant, he felt on edge and vigilant. He was fearful of embarrassing himself by saying something stupid. Like many people with SAD, he reported that social anxiety had been noticeable even when he was a child. Now that he didn't have alcohol to self-medicate, he claimed that the painful shyness of his youth had returned after 40 years.

With John, I took a cognitive behavioral approach and used some of the treatment ideas in the "Treatment Tips" section. I started by educating him on how to eradicate the ANTS (automatic negative thoughts) by identifying his cognitive distortions, using handouts such as "Problematic Thinking" (Handout 2.2) and "Examples of Depression- and Anxiety-Producing Cognitive Distortions" (Handout 2.3). As I helped him get to the bottom of his irrational thoughts, he was able to increasingly gain control over his anxiety.

This chapter on anxiety builds on the first chapter about stress. After all, unmanageable stress is a cornerstone of anxiety. However, we learned in the last chapter that if stress is managed, it can be motivating and exhilarating, and that in any case, stress is necessary for a well-balanced life. The age-old dilemma is how to help your clients contain worry and anxiety so that it works for them and motivates rather than debilitates them. In this chapter, we will focus on solutions that you can offer your clients to help them calm down from an anxious state. There are no one-size-fits all approaches. What works for one client might not work for another, so having many tools in your therapeutic toolbox is essential. This chapter provides a variety of mindfulness-based, acceptance-based, and cognitive behavioral strategies to help your clients manage their anxiety.

It is important to be flexible in trying various approaches. When one technique doesn't work, try another; solution-oriented therapists will have many tools in their toolbox to use when one tool does not work. Remind your client that anxiety is a curable problem, and that only by addressing it and not avoiding it will you be able to arrive at solutions together. It is important to help clients see that anxiety is something to learn from and manage, not something to push away and resist facing. Addressing anxiety is the only way to master it; otherwise, anxiety is allowed to be the master. I offer my clients this rule of thumb: *What you resist will persist.*

Treatment Tips

In this section, I offer a variety of treatment techniques from Cognitive Behavior Therapy (CBT) and third-wave psychotherapy approaches, characterized by mindfulness and acceptance practices. Having an array of solution-oriented approaches in your therapeutic toolbox will allow you to offer your clients many opportunities to master their anxiety.

With the availability of numerous self-help books and other resources for practitioners on how to reduce anxiety and panic, these techniques by no means constitute an exhaustive list. However, I personally have found these tips useful, and they have appeared time and time again in many of the most popular treatment handbooks from various CBT practitioners. Many of the following strategies have also withstood various research studies on their effectiveness. Fortunately, there are many types of techniques that offer treatment tools to your anxiety treatment toolbox. Every client comes with his or her own unique set of needs, skills, and issues, and having many techniques to offer them will provide many opportunities for success.

To help clients face their anxiety in a productive way, we often need to first educate them about anxiety. "Common Myths About Anxiety" (Handout 2.1) is a good way to begin doing that. In this section, I offer additional ways of beginning to lay a foundation of what anxiety is with clients, using a few short mini-lessons from CBT and third-wave approaches, followed by practical treatment strategies on how to master anxiety from both major areas. I use treatment tools from various approaches, such as CBT, Dialectical Behavior Therapy (DBT), Acceptance and Commitment Therapy (ACT), and Mindfulness-Based Cognitive Therapy (MBCT), to fill up my therapeutic toolbox. The following treatment tips are examples of practices from various treatment modalities.

☑ *Mini-Lesson: Welcoming Anxiety to Motivate, Not Debilitate*

Teaching clients that anxiety—just like stress—can be their friend instead of their foe will already make them less anxious! When clients learn that anxiety can serve to motivate rather than debilitate, they will be more likely to learn from it rather than to avoid it. All too often, we get anxious over being anxious, and after a while it's hard to know what the real problem is—the reason we initially got anxious, or the anxiety over being anxious. An effective metaphor I use with my clients is the "low-fuel" warning on a car. When the gaslight turns on, we are reminded that the gas level is low and that the car needs refueling. Likewise, we get anxious when there is something we need to pay attention to—otherwise, we will run out of "gas"! We need worry and anxiety to keep ourselves safe and productive in order to run on all cylinders!

Consider the following:

- If we didn't worry, we might very well drink alcohol and drive.
- If we didn't have anxiety about our job performance, we might end up slacking off and not being well prepared for an important meeting presentation.
- If we didn't worry that we could lose our jobs, we might take extra vacation days than allotted or not work our normal workweek, causing us to get fired.
- If we weren't anxious about taking safety precautions when driving a car or riding a bike, we wouldn't be defensive enough to avoid accidents.
- If we weren't anxious on a ski slope, we might overestimate our abilities, causing accidents and collisions.
- If we weren't anxious about our children's safety, we might not be as vigilant in caring for them.
- If we weren't anxious about performing in a play, concert, or competition, we wouldn't rehearse as much and would be less prepared.

In sum, anxiety within limits can be motivating and ensures our safety and our successes. It's when anxiety controls our mind, rather than our mind controlling the anxiety, that the nervous and anxious thoughts pull us down rather than lift us up.

☑ Mini-Lesson: Understanding the Fight-or-Flight Response

To help our clients face their anxiety, it is helpful to teach them that anxiety is actually adaptive and necessary for survival. A short lesson on the normal physiological reaction to threat—the fight-or-flight response —will help your clients see the importance of learning from the warning signs our anxiety gives us. In the fight-or-flight response, animals as well as humans release hormones and produce a chemical reaction when danger is perceived. This involves an increase in tension in the sympathetic nervous system, which gears up the body to flee or fight to ward off danger. The fight-or-flight response is known largely as being the first stage of the normal reaction to stress: the General Adaptation Syndrome. An increase in anxiety results in physical manifestations such as higher metabolism, higher blood pressure, greater perspiration, more rapid breathing, and a faster heart rate. From the stance of evolution, this response is necessary for individual and species survival. Without this physiological response to a stressor in the environment, animals, including humans, would not be able to protect themselves from imminent danger. Thus, it is adaptive to have this stress response, and educating your clients about the importance of not fighting their reactions, but learning from them, will be quite helpful.

The problem comes when this fight-or-flight response is on overdrive and keeps a person in a state of high alert, making it difficult from him or her to calm back down and relax when imminent danger has subsided. This overdrive reaction leads to tensions, nervousness, and a generalized state of anxiety, severely handicapping an individual's sense of well-being and mental clarity.

☑ Mini-Lesson: Introducing Mindfulness

All of the third-wave modalities emphasize the importance of using mindfulness techniques to treat panic and anxiety. Contrary to what many people think, mindfulness is not emptying your mind and "spacing out." It is not even necessarily relaxing or being calm. Rather, it is an act of creating space between one's thoughts and one's sense of self. It is actually a skills-based practice for learning how to be more in control of your mind so that you are more self-aware and *present*, while suspending the common judgments that often crowd our inner thoughts. With mindfulness practice, you become a witness to those disturbing thoughts, looking *at* them objectively instead of *from* them.

45

This is a very important distinction. When your clients look *from* their thoughts, they don't have the perspective and objectivity to be non-judgmental and descriptive about them. Thus, they end up believing very illogical conclusions that result in disturbing and extremely negative emotions, which in turn end up often causing disturbing behavioral reactions. On the other hand, when you teach your clients to look *at* their thoughts, they learn the skills to observe them without personalizing them, and to distance themselves from only irrational conclusions they might make. Therefore, disturbing and intense emotional reactions do not result, and clients learn valuable skills for distancing themselves from overwhelming anxiety while at the same time attending to the anxiety without denying or running away from it.

Mindfulness therapist and author Terry Fralich (2013) describes this shift into present awareness as like being a *witness* to your thoughts. This takes the power away from your inner critic, which is full of automatic judgments that interfere with self-love and self-compassion. As we become more objectively mindful of our automatic negative thoughts about others and ourselves, we develop more compassion and loving-kindness toward others and ourselves.

As you can see from this difference above, the main criterion for mindfulness practice is non-judgmental awareness, not the typical meditation-style practice that has often been confused with acceptance- and mindfulness-based treatment strategies. Although meditation can be an example of a mindfulness exercise, mindfulness practice does not mean that you have to be quiet, have your eyes closed, and stay calm. Rather, mindfulness techniques require only that you are focused on the present and engaged in the moment, in whatever you are doing. Fralich (2013) offers some sample self-affirming phrases to focus on while practicing the art of nonjudgmental mindfulness:

"I am glad I noticed my inner critic."
"It gives me a chance to be kind and gentle to myself."
"May I feel kind to myself."
"May I feel the warmth of my being."

"May I connect with the goodness of my true nature."
"May I feel the love that connects everyone and everything."

In summary, mindfulness refers to nonjudgmental self-awareness. It is a practice for everyday life, not one that shuts out the world and isolates us. Rather, mindfulness helps us fully engage in what we are doing in the moment. One of the most common mindfulness practices suggested by third-wave approaches is making mindfulness part of your everyday routine. With this in mind, encourage your clients to try to be more aware and observant in everything they do: brushing their teeth, getting dressed, eating, washing dishes, driving to work, walking from their car, listening to music, and so on. For example, in the case of taking a shower, encourage your clients to notice the smell of the soap, the feel of the shampoo, the sensation of water spraying on their body, the way the light is reflected in the room, the feel of the towel as they dry off. While this is happening, they can also be aware of their thoughts coming and going—observing them but detaching from them so as to develop the ability to gain a rational perspective, free of distortions and negative judgments that are regarded as fact.

☑ Activity: Daily Records and Anxiety Logs

One of the cornerstones of the treatment of anxiety in all CBT and third-wave practices is the use of logs, journals, and diaries to track thoughts, feelings, and behaviors. Very few client symptoms are as conducive to the use of these resources as anxiety, and the "Handouts" section of this chapter provides templates you can use with your clients that encompass some of the major elements in most logs. In addition, the Recommended Resources section provides links to helpful web resources that offer daily logs as well as many other worksheets. Many of these materials can be downloaded and reproduced for your clients, with some available only through purchase, such as those on the Beck Institute site and David Burns's site. I have also included the resource sites for some of the most influential thought leaders in the field of counseling today, so that you can access a variety of inventories, tests, and worksheets not included in this book.

In the "Handouts" section, I have provided worksheets and logs to help clients track and manage their anxiety. "Analyzing Anxiety: Daily Log" (Handout 2.4) is a blank worksheet, and "Analyzing Anxiety: Daily Log Completed" (Handout 2.5) is a completed model worksheet. These offer clients opportunities to track their anxious thoughts, feelings, and behaviors, while the "Daily or Weekly Anxiety Summary Log" (Handout 2.6) and "Weekly Anxiety Record" (Handout 2.7) offers variations of basic thought logs to help clients manage their anxiety.

Effective solution-oriented treatment includes thought records, worksheets, and logs so that clients can employ the self-help strategies they learn between sessions. All modalities of CBT and third-wave approaches incorporate a multitude of self-help assignments to structure your client's practice between sessions. Although daily practice log entries are ideal, for most clients daily homework is not realistic, and often with my clients I expect just a few entries on a relevant worksheet for the week. The timing will depend on the motivation of the client, the degree of severity of the problem, and what phase of treatment the client is in. Since clients are often not used to this type of "homework" at the beginning of therapy and are just learning the general concepts of treatment, I start slowly so as not to overwhelm them with too many expectations. Especially when working with anxious clients, you don't want to set up a situation where they feel more anxious! I learned this from one client who confided in me that she'd had to go online to find out how to fill in the logs, as separating thoughts, feelings, and behaviors was not as easy for her as I assumed it would be.

The common element among the various types of logs is that they encourage clients to pay regular attention to the development of life coping skills and provide a way to track them. Most of them prompt clients to separate their thoughts from their feelings or to rate the degree of their belief or the degree of their anxiety for each entry, which highlights the relative weight, or importance, clients place on that entry. This also helps clients realize that even if they are anxious, it is not a black-and-white issue, and that the degree of their anxiety is more manageable and more under their control than they might have realized. This focus on degree of belief or anxiety originated in the concept of SUDS, or subjective units of distress, a term coined in 1969 by behaviorist Joseph Wolpe. The scaling of SUDS is often still used today in many tracking logs and behavioral diaries, especially in the case of anxiety, for which the SUDS scale was designed.

☑ Activity: Use the Power of Bibliotherapy

It is not a coincidence that bibliotherapy has the word *therapy* in it. Reading books will reinforce what clients have learned in session, and will help them use self-help avenues to develop the psychoeducational skills they need to master their anxiety. Just as a music student needs to practice playing music between sessions, your clients won't be able to incorporate lessons learned in session unless they read on their own and reinforce their learning with practice using handouts and worksheets to build their skills. There are numerous self-help books you can recommend that will dovetail nicely with what your clients learn in therapy, and they can fast-forward alleviation of anxiety symptoms.

There are many studies that point to the effectiveness of bibliotherapy. In his *Feeling Good Handbook* (1999), David Burns cites an important study he did with potential clients who were on a waiting list to be seen for therapy at Pennsylvania Hospital in Philadelphia in the 1990s. The prospective patients on the waiting list were split up into two groups—one that received David Burns's *Feeling Good Handbook* while waiting to get their first appointment, and one that received no book. The waiting-list clients who received a copy of the handbook improved much more than the waiting-list clients who did not receive a copy. In fact, quite a few members of the former group reported that their symptoms of depression and anxiety had subsided enough that they no longer needed an appointment. Even Albert Ellis, in his book *How to Control Your Anxiety Before It Controls You* (1998), claimed that many people benefitted just as much from reading his pamphlets as they did from being in psychotherapy with him.

The "Recommended Resources" section in this chapter lists some of my favorite self-help books for overcoming anxiety, which all are "hands-on" and psychoeducational in nature. Each of the books offers many practical skill-building activities and self-help assignments, which ideally will be executed in conjunction with therapy. By going over self-help assignments found in the books in session, you can help clients become more active in their quest to overcome their anxiety.

☑ ACT Techniques: Cognitive Defusion Visualizations

One of the most important terms to teach your clients as they learn mindfulness strategies is the ACT term *cognitive defusion*, which entails looking at thoughts in a new way. *Cognitive fusion* refers to being *fused* with your thoughts so that there is no separation, leading to an unquestioning acceptance of distorted thinking. Those thoughts become just like reality, and if our clients are unable to separate themselves from their anxiety-ridden thoughts, they become fused with their anxiety and can not gain an objective distance from it.

In *cognitive defusion*, clients are taught to distance themselves from debilitating and negative thoughts. This key mindfulness concept makes use of various visualization practices that help clients distance themselves from their thoughts, and consequently from their feelings and reactions, developing an "observing head." The underlying rationale of this concept is that too much suffering is caused by overidentification with and attachment to disturbing thoughts, which end up getting entangled in a web of anxiety and distortions. Regular practice of *cognitive defusion* leads to better objectivity and more distance from those disturbing reactions. Teach your clients the difference between observing their thoughts and identifying with them as part of themselves. That way, your clients can detach and disentangle themselves from the disturbing thoughts that cause so much anxiety and suffering.

Cognitive defusion is one of the core self-help techniques of Acceptance and Commitment Therapy. When we think in more objective terms, we can say, "I am having the thought that I am a loser" rather than thinking and believing that "I am a loser." The first option is factual, dispassionate, and informative, while the second one is irrationally subjective and states a thought as if it were a fact. It is also helpful to label the thoughts—for instance, "my thought that I am unlovable" is an example of a distorted perception."

The following are some cognitive defusion visualizations:

Imagining leaves on a floating stream. This is one of the most popular mindfulness practices used in ACT and MBCT to cope with anxious thoughts. Have your clients imagine leaves floating on a stream. Then have them imagine that each disturbing thought is placed on a leaf, outside their head, and encourage them to watch those thoughts float away in all different directions and disappear. (For a terrific detailed description of this technique, see the reference by Harris, 2009.)

Watching your thoughts on a computer screen. Using the image of a computer screen, suggest to your clients to watch their thoughts like a ticker tape going across the screen. This will help them to distance themselves from them rather than identify with them.

Imagine balloons drifting away. Have your clients imagine holding a whole cluster of balloons, each with an anxious thought written on it or on a piece of paper inside of it. Then suggest to them to imagine themselves letting go and watching the balloons fly away and disappear into thin air.

Watching your thoughts on a movie screen. My clients have found it quite helpful to distance themselves from their anxious thoughts by imagining that they are sitting in the audience of a movie theater, watching their actions and thoughts on the screen. Imagining themselves in the back row of the theater will help them even more distance themselves from any disturbing thoughts. Remind them that movies stretch the truth to make good stories. With his in mind, have them look *at* their thoughts, rather than *from* them. If they are experiencing persistant disturbing thoughts, suggest to them that they distance from them by rephrasing them and putting the new wording on the movie screen—for example, "I am watching myself express fear of fainting from anxiety" rather than "I am going to faint from anxiety."

☑ *Mindfulness Techniques: Relaxation and Guided Imagery*

DBT, ACT, and MBCT all stress the importance of relaxing the body as well as the mind. MBCT, for example, has clients regularly practice a body scan, in which they focus progressively on sensations of various parts of their body systematically. There is no shortage of variations of relaxation and visualization exercises, the rationale being that the mind and body both need to work well together. Especially in the case of panic, when physiological reactions are very powerful, paying attention to breathing and bodily sensation can help control anxiety. Edmund Bourne, author of the popular Anxiety and Phobia Workbook (1990), emphasizes the importance of taking care of your body as a prerequisite to calming your anxiety. Paying attention to good nutrition, eliminating or minimizing caffeine intake, and getting regular exercise are just some of the recommendations he makes in his book to help readers conquer their anxiety. His point is that focusing on the mind will not be enough, since anxiety and phobic reactions entail so many physical reactions.

It is important to keep in mind that third-wave theorists do not reject the cognitive behavior approach—far from it. Rather, they include the cognitive orientation in their approaches, and have added to it with focus on the present-centered awareness practices of acceptance and mindfulness.

☑ *CBT Technique: Eradicate the ANTS*

CBT theorists often refer to "automatic negative thoughts" using a catchy title: *ANTS*. Eradicating the ANTS in your head often requires not only education, but also written exercises designed to help in identifying the ANTS. These worksheets are important for clients to use between sessions to practice their skills. In session, to catch some ANTS from clients, I often write them down as they are talking, and then read back to them what they said. I then show the clients how to replace the ANTS with more rational thoughts. Not only is this a very effective technique in the session itself, but it also models for the client what to do between sessions, setting an example of how to do "thought catching" in every-day life. Whether they fill out a log or write down their thoughts on notecards or paper, clients benefit from writing out their ANTS and challenging them with healthier, more objective alternatives.

☑ *CBT Technique: Labeling and Categorizing Your Thoughts*

One essential practice of all CBT theorists is that of identifying and labeling cognitive distortions. A checklist of cognitive distortions has been developed by Aaron Beck and popularized by self-help guru David Burns. Various worksheets and handouts by CBT theorists help clients categorize their negative and irrational thoughts, helping them pinpoint the type of cognitive error they are making. The following are a sampling of some of the cognitive errors that are the mainstay of CBT theorists' logs and worksheets, including Burns's popular Daily Mood Log. Holding on to these type of cognitive distortions can prove paralyzing, and thoughts like these are at the root of anxiety. Handout 2.3 ("Examples of Depression- and Anxiety- Producing Cognitive Distortions") can be used frequently by your client to identify the types of cognitive distortions to which they are prone. It is one thing for them to know that they have irrational thoughts, but another to know the *type* of thinking error they are experiencing. Identifying the type of cognitive distortion they are experiencing can help them see patterns in their misperceptions so that they are more likely to change their distorted cognitive filters. Identifying the type of cognitive distortions, also known as thinking errors, helps clients look at their problematic thinking in a more objective manner.

This is just a small sampling of cognitive distortions that are particularly common in symptoms of Anxiety. See Handout 2.3 for a more in-depth list.

- *All-or-nothing thinking.* You see things as all bad or all good, and thus blow them out of proportion. Instead of seeing your anxiety as *inconvenient* or *difficult*, you see it in black-and-white terms such as *horrible* and *awful*.
  Example: "It would be horrible if I stumbled on my words!"
- *Personalization.* You assume you are at fault or are inadequate.
  Example: "She seems bored—she must hate talking to me!"

- *Labeling.* You label yourself in a derogatory way if you make a mistake or fail.
  Example: "I failed; therefore, I'm a failure."
- *Fortune telling.* You predict negative outcomes as if they were fact.
  Example: "My boss will be mad if I ask too many questions and she'll think I'm lame."
- *"Shoulding."* You think in inflexible ways, using words like *must* and *should*, limiting flexible and compassionate thinking and fueling even more anxiety.
  Example: "I shouldn't make mistakes, and I must be liked by everyone."

☑ CBT Technique: The Experimental Technique

When clients blow out of proportion how awful or catastrophic something will be, have them test the validity of their assumptions by conducting experiments between sessions. For example, a socially anxious student who thinks that none of his classmates want to talk with him can try to start conversations before or after class and report back to you how people actually respond.

☑ CBT Technique: Downward or Vertical Arrow Technique

This is a core technique in CBT intervention, popularized by both Beck and Burns, to get to the self-defeating core beliefs that are the source of a considerable amount of anxiety.

Here is an example of how I used this technique with a client of mine who was extremely anxious about meeting a group of college friends:

Client:	Therapist:
"I am afraid to go to my college reunion."	
	"Why would that be a problem? Why would that bother you?"
↓	
"They would be so surprised at how fat I am."	

"Why would that be a problem?
Why would that bother you?"

↓

"Because they will pity me."

"Why would that be a problem?
Why would that bother you?"

↓

"They will see that my life never
amounted to anything."

"Why would that be a problem?
Why would that bother you?"

↓

Core belief: "Because I am a loser
and don't want to be reminded of
that."

This vertical arrow technique helped me examine with my client her core beliefs about being a disappointment and a loser. We were able to identify the cognitive distortions of fortune telling, labeling, personalization, and all-or-nothing thinking. After we used this model in session, my client was able to practice this technique between sessions, which helped her to identify the roots of her anxiety and challenge her basic assumptions that had faulty logic.

Burns uses the downward arrow technique to elicit core beliefs, often following them with the "What if?" and feared fantasy techniques, described in the next two tips.

☑ CBT Technique: The "What if?" Technique

After using the downward arrow technique and uncovering the core beliefs at the root of his clients' anxiety, Burns often uses the "What if?" technique. To carry out this technique, he merely asks, "What if this were true?" in response to his clients' irrational anxieties. Clients often answer with thoughts such as "I couldn't stand it!" "I would die!" or "I wouldn't be able to handle it!" No wonder this type of thinking leads to significant and paralyzing anxiety! The "What if?" technique uncovers the irrational fantasies that lead to extreme anxiety.

Thirty-eight-year-old Linda was starting a new job and was very anxious about making mistakes and "failing." Every time she got an email from her boss (who worked remotely), her anxiety would be overwhelming, and it would take her minutes to have the courage to open the email. She was afraid he would find a mistake and be upset with her. She read between the lines in his emails, often reading annoyance about her into them. Using the "What if?" technique in session, I asked her what she feared, and her response was that she was afraid her boss would criticize her and maybe even fire her. She kept being afraid he would express his displeasure. I asked her, "What if that were true?" to each of her stated fears of how her boss might react. Getting to the bottom of her fears, she realized she was most fearful of losing her job and not being able to provide a stable life for her children, as her parents had been unable to do for her. She was afraid of losing her home, which objectively was very unrealistic since her husband also had a very good income and a lot of job security.

Even though this technique was somewhat effective, her deep-seated fears of being like her parents and not providing a stable life for her children still emotionally paralyzed her. My next step was to use the feared fantasy technique.

☑ CBT Technique: Feared Fantasy

With my client Linda, I followed the "What If?" technique with the even more thought-provoking feared fantasy technique. This involves carrying the fantasy that you fear to the extreme, even to the point of absurdity. Clients either can write down the words of the critic in their feared fantasy, or they can role-play with the therapist their worst, most exaggerated fears.

I asked Linda to explore her worst fantasies and what she would imagine her boss might say (conjuring up almost a cartoon image). She admitted that her worst fantasy was having her boss find out she was stupid and be so disgusted with her inability to "catch on" that he fired her. Her feared fantasy did not stop there. She then imagined that she was homeless, her husband and children, drifting from place to place, even worse than in her own unstable youth. I asked her to exaggerate the fear and to fantasize herself and her husband living in squalor or a homeless shelter, unable to provide for their children. Her fantasies of her boss telling her that she was the most stupid employee that he ever had, leading eventually to her being thrown out of her home, at first made my client more anxious, but as we explored each fantasy in detail, she began to see the absurdity of her fears and calmed down. She even laughed about some of the images. By allowing herself to go along with her "feared fantasy," she was no longer immobilized by her hidden fears. Using this technique, she realized just how far fetched her scenario was, and she began to relax and be less fearful about getting emails from her boss. Following the "What if" technique with the feared fantasy technique proved to be very effective in jarring persistent and deep seated anxious thoughts, using the element of the absurd.

☑ CBT Technique: Cost/Benefit Analysis

One of the common behavioral interventions used by many CBT and DBT practitioners is analysis of the benefits and costs of having a certain belief, anxiety, or behavior. Writing down the advantages and disadvantages of having, for example, certain anxious beliefs, helps clients understand the reinforcement that might come as a result of their fear. For example, take the example of a college age client who does not ask out a classmate for a date for fear he will be rejected. One advantage is that he doesn't have to face rejection and feel embarrassed, but a strong disadvantage is that he is lonely and is preventing himself from having a relationship. Having clients fill out a cost/benefit analysis homework sheet, rating from 1–100 the strength of their conviction for each side, helps them become more objective and matter-of-fact about their anxieties.

☑ Behavioral and CBT Techniques: Exposure

Some of the oldest forms of behavior therapy in treating anxiety are the exposure techniques of gradual exposure, flooding, and systematic desensitization. Meeting your fears and anxieties by either imagining them or actually immersing yourself in them is not for the faint of heart, but might offer hope for highly resistant anxieties. Two major exposure techniques are flooding and systematic desensitization.

FLOODING

Flooding is a behavioral technique in which anxiety disorders such as phobias are treated by exposure to the feared stimulus. Using classical and operant-conditioning techniques, clients immerse themselves in the thing they fear.

Psychiatrist Joseph Wolpe (1990) carried out an experiment that demonstrated flooding. He had a young female client who was scared of cars, and he drove her around in his car for a few hours. This cured her of her phobia of going into cars! Albert Ellis informally used the flooding technique on himself when he was 19. Painfully shy and afraid of approaching women, he forced himself to approach 100 women at the New York Botanical Garden. Although he never got a date with any of those 100 women, he reported that facing his fears made him much less anxious about going up to women and talking, and his fear of approaching women was cured.

Flooding is sometimes used in attempting to cure specific phobias. For example, using flooding to treat a phobia of going in an elevator would entail going in an elevator, perhaps with a therapist, family member, or friend. However, this can often be traumatic for clients, so gradual exposure and systematic desensitization are preferred choices of treatment to avoid further traumatization.

GRADUAL EXPOSURE

This anxiety-busting technique is a more relaxed type of flooding that takes place over time, and thus is less intense and potentially traumatic than flooding. In this technique, a hierarchy of anxiety-producing fears are rated from least anxiety provoking to most anxiety provoking.

In Ellis's case, instead of having him approach women cold turkey, the gradual exposure technique would have allowed him to break his fears into smaller goals, beginning with a less fearful situation, such as sitting on a bench at the gardens and watching women walk by. For the next step, he would just smile when they walked by. Other smaller steps might include talking to other men or women with young babies, just to get comfortable with talking to other people at the Botanical Garden. Little by little, he would master the small steps to approaching women, and eventually he would work up to asking them for a date.

SYSTEMATIC DESENSITIZATION

Initially developed by behaviorist Joseph Wolpe, systematic desensitization is a time-tested method of mastering anxiety and helping clients overcome strong fears, pairing deep breathing and relaxation techniques with a hierarchy of feared events that are first introduced in the office and then in real life.

Twenty-two-year-old Jan, one of my very first clients over 35 years ago, had a phobia of eating in front of others. This was at about the time that fast food was just becoming popular, and the first McDonalds had just come to town. Using relaxation methods—specifically, having her systematically relax different parts of her body (similar to MBCT's body scan, developed years later)—I had her perform small steps in a hierarchy of feared events. First she imagined herself driving by the McDonald's, sitting in the parking lot, running in and ordering a meal, and eating in her car. She then carried out these steps in real life, to the point where she actually ordered a meal at McDonald's and sat in the restaurant to eat!

A Toolkit of Metaphors for Treating Anxiety

Metaphorical objects to assemble in your clients' "worry-free toolkit" can serve as valuable reminders throughout the day, to help them to manage their anxiety. Having objects in your office or bringing them to a group session offers many opportunities to help clients develop mastery over their anxiety. Objects also provide opportunities to use humor to help lighten the anxious mood.

For larger items that can't fit into a small bag, you can have notecards on hand so clients can draw their own, or for a group activity, you can provide magazines for clients to cut pictures out that represent a metaphor for combatting anxiety.

The following are examples of the anxiety toolkit:

Beach ball. Imagine a beach ball being pushed into a body of water—it keeps popping up! This represents what happens to our anxious thoughts when we keep trying to suppress them. This is a very convincing metaphor regarding the importance of giving up resistance to our anxiety by employing the strategies of acceptance and mindfulness.

Thought train. This ACT metaphor represents the train of our thoughts. We can imagine watching the train from above with each section of the train having written on it an anxious thought—we can watch it without jumping aboard. This is an example of cognitive defusion.

Bendable figure. Staying flexible helps alleviate anxiety.

Spiral cooking coil whisk. A spiral whisk reminds us that our anxieties can spiral out of control, which will keep us spiraling downward.

Post-it note or file card with a picture of a rocking chair. Write reminders and sayings, such as, "Worry is like a rocking chair—no matter how much you rock, you never get anywhere!"

Sand timer. Give yourself a worry time—and once the time is up, leave your worries until you decide to have another worry session. For working with groups, I purchase sand timers in bulk at online distributors to give out in meetings to give clients a tangible reminder to bring home of how to control worry.

Can you and your clients add to this toolkit?

Therapeutic Takeaways

☑ Teach your clients that anxiety is adaptive and important for our physical and emotional survival. Just like stress, anxiety can be productive if it is managed.

☑ Anxiety disorders affect one fifth of the population, and are a major reason that clients seek counseling. Some of the most common anxiety disorders are generalized anxiety disorder, posttraumatic stress disorder, panic, specific phobias, and social anxiety disorder.

☑ Use mindfulness visualizations that incorporate cognitive defusion with your anxious clients, teaching them how to be less judgmental, more accepting, and more present focused, so that they can learn to look *at* their thoughts instead of *from* their thoughts.

☑ Successful treatment of anxiety entails a mind-body approach. Relaxation exercises help to calm the body as well as the mind.

☑ Cognitive treatment for anxiety includes a mix of imagery and actual practice in which clients test out their predictions and anxieties in a variety of ways. There are many CBT strategies that help clients identify their cognitive distortions and core irrational beliefs, which helps lessen their anxiety. A wealth of cognitive techniques can offer you as a clinician many tools for your therapeutic toolbox—no one technique fits everybody.

☑ Bibliotherapy, self-help worksheets, and logs and diaries all give clients opportunities to practice the skills they have learned in session. Successful treatment makes use of these resources for between-session strategies.

Handouts

The following worksheets will help your clients manage anxiety. As a general guideline, handouts and assignments are given to your clients at the end of the session. Make sure you leave ample time to go over how you want your client to use the selected handout.

When assignments are given out, it is important to follow up with your clients at the beginning of the next session. Going over homework is an essential aspect of being a solution-oriented therapist.

Note: All handouts in the book are available for download on my website by following the link below: http://www.belmontwellness.com/ultimate-solution-handouts/

Handout 2.1: Common Myths About Anxiety

Myth 1: Anxiety and fear are generally interchangeable.

Fear and anxiety often trigger similar physiological responses, but they are different in terms of their origins. Anxiety is a response to a vague threat, while fear is a response to a known threat. For example, walking on a dark city street can understandably bring about anxiety because of all the unknowns lurking in the dark, whereas actual fear might occur if you saw or sensed a large man walking toward you in the dark. We need these reactions to keep us vigilant and safe.

Myth 2: Anxiety is bad for you.

We need the fight-or-flight response to survive, and thus anxiety is quite adaptive. Anxiety can be likened to a low-fuel warning light on your car's dashboard. Just as the gas light warns you that you are running close to empty and need to refuel, anxiety alerts you to issues that need attention so that you can achieve insights and emotionally refuel and thus move forward in your life.

Myth 3: It is best to avoid anxiety and not give in to it.

The more you fight anxiety, the more you will be caught in its grips. The founder of Acceptance and Commitment Therapy (ACT), Steven Hayes, used the image of the finger trap carnival toy to demonstrate what happens when you fight anxiety rather than accept it. Only when you give up pulling and resisting will you be able to get out of the trap.

Myth 4: If you have an anxiety disorder, it is best to avoid stressful situations.

To the contrary, cognitive behavior therapists such as Aaron Beck and David Burns actually use techniques such as "flooding" and "exposure" to aid their clients in conquering anxiety. Using these techniques, we can confront our worst fears, either in reality or in their imagination. The underlying premise is that avoiding and escaping anxiety-provoking thoughts only makes them increase and gives them too much power. Contrary to popular belief and our common instinctual behaviors, avoidance of anxiety actually increases levels of anxiety.

Myth 5: Although anxiety is common, anxiety disorders are not.

Research studies, including those from the National Institute of Mental Health, have shown that anxiety disorders affect almost 1 out of 5 people at some point in their lives. Some of the most common types of anxiety disorders, affecting millions, are phobias, social phobias, social anxiety, generalized anxiety disorder, and panic disorder.

The Anxiety Solution

Handout 2.2: Problematic Thinking

Notice the words in bold—they are inflexible, blown out of proportion, or illogical, or they represent all-or-nothing thinking. These kinds of
statements lead to anxiety.

1. I **can't** stand it!
2. It is **terrible** that things go **wrong**!
3. He **shouldn't** be that way!
4. I **hate** being criticized!
5. They **should** listen to me!
6. I **can't** change what I think!
7. It's **terrible** to be wrong!
8. I **should** be able to control my kids' behavior!
9. I **can't** forgive them/myself!
10. He makes me **nuts**!
11. It **drives me crazy**!
12. He **ruined** my life!
13. Things are **hopeless**!
14. It's **awful**!
15. It's my **fault** she's like that!
16. My childhood **always** affects me!
17. She **made me** feel that way!
18. I **can't** control my feelings!
19. I **can't** help the way I act!
20. He **always** does that!

Do you notice any phrases that relate to you? Write them or other
problematic thoughts below and change them into healthier thoughts.

Problematic Thinking	Healthy Thinking
Example: She **made me** feel that way!	She cannot control my feelings. Rather, I felt that way when she said that.
_____	_____
_____	_____
_____	_____
_____	_____

Handout 2.3: Examples of Depression and Anxiety-Producing Cognitive Distortions

The following are some cognitive distortions that are at the root of anxiety based on the work of CBT pioneers Aaron Beck and David Burns:

1. *ALL-OR-NOTHING THINKING:* You see things in black-and-white categories. If you make a mistake, you might think that you "failed" or are a "failure."
2. *OVERGENERALIZATION:* You generalize from a specific. You think in absolutes, like *always* and *never*, and see a single negative event as a never-ending pattern.
3. *MENTAL FILTER:* You pick out a single negative event and dwell on it, like a drop of ink that discolors a whole glass of water.
4. *MAGNIFICATION or MINIMIZATION:* You either blow things out of proportion or deny that something is a problem when it is. Examples: *"I am the worst mother ever"* or *"It's nothing—no big deal"* (when it really is a big deal to you).
5. *"SHOULD" STATEMENTS:* You have preconceived ideas about how you and other people "should" be. Judgmental and unforgiving expectations create a lot of anxiety.
6. *PERSONALIZATION:* You are self-conscious and think things are about you when that is just your interpretation. When someone behaves negatively, you think that that behavior is a response to you, and then blame yourself.
7. *PLAYING THE COMPARISON GAME:* You compare yourself to others and feel the need to keep up with or outshine others to feel good about yourself. Example: "He is so much smarter than me; I'm stupid."
8. *FORTUNE TELLING:* You think that you can predict the future, and you convince yourself that bad things will happen. Example: "I will always have these problems!"
9. *LABELING:* You label yourself or others by terms such as *lazy, fat, stupid, loser,* and *jerk,* stating them as if they were facts. A label becomes an erroneous evaluation of self-worth.

Now, write some examples of your own anxiety-producing thoughts in the left column. In the right-hand column, identify the types of distortions for each thought.

Irrational Thoughts	Cognitive Distortions
Example: I am a loser and always will be	Labeling, fortune telling, all-or-nothing thinking
_____	_____
_____	_____
_____	_____
_____	_____
_____	_____
_____	_____
_____	_____

Handout 2.4: Analyzing Anxiety: Daily Log

Anxiety-Triggering Event	
Negative Emotions	Positive Emotions
Strength of Negative Emotions 1 2 3 4 5 6 7 8 9 10 Low High	Strength of Positive Emotions 1 2 3 4 5 6 7 8 9 10 Low High
Identify Negative Anxious Beliefs	Challenge With Positive Beliefs
Type of Cognitive Distortion	Response to Cognitive Distortion
Certainty of Your Beliefs _____ 1 2 3 4 5 6 7 8 9 10 Low High	Certainty of Your Beliefs _____ 1 2 3 4 5 6 7 8 9 10 Low High
Unhealthy Reactions	Healthy Reactions
Cost/Benefit Analysis: Unhealthy Coping	Cost/Benefit Analysis: Healthy Coping
My Conclusions and Goals	

Handout 2.5: Analyzing Anxiety: Daily Log Completed

Anxiety-Triggering Event	
Fear of rejection in anticipation of going to a singles mixer	
Negative Emotions Anxiety	**Positive Emotions** Excitement over possibly meeting someone
Strength of Negative Emotions _____X_____ 1 2 3 4 5 6 7 8 9 10 Low High	**Strength of Positive Emotions** _____X_____ 1 2 3 4 5 6 7 8 9 10 Low High
Identify Negative Anxious Beliefs Women don't notice me. There will be much better people than me there. What if no one bothers with me?	**Challenge With Positive Beliefs** Even if I am ignored, that doesn't take away my self-worth. I am proud of myself for trying to meet someone.
Type of Cognitive Distortion Comparison game, all or nothing things.	**Response to Cognitive Distortion** I will not compare myself with others or exaggerate.
Certainty of Your Beliefs _____X_____ 1 2 3 4 5 6 7 8 9 10 Low High	**Certainty of Your Beliefs** _____X____ 1 2 3 4 5 6 7 8 9 10 Low High
Unhealthy Reactions Going to the singles mixer and leaving right away Staying to myself, not initiating talking	**Healthy Reactions** Initiating conversation Trying to practice assertive skills I learned
Cost/Benefit Analysis: Unhealthy Coping Costs: I will be alone and lonely and not give myself a chance to meet someone	**Cost/Benefit Analysis: Healthy Coping** Benefits: I will be safe and protect myself from humiliation and rejection.
My Conclusions and Goals	
I am committed to continuing to try and practice, and I will make a realistic goal for this year to improve my assertiveness.	

Handout 2.6: Daily or Weekly Anxiety Summary Log

Date(s): _____

1. Anxiety-provoking events

_____

_____

2. Emotional responses

_____

_____

3. Degree of anxiety   LOW 1 2 3 4 5 6 7 8 9 10 HIGH

4. Unhealthy thoughts

_____

_____

Certainty of beliefs   LOW 1 2 3 4 5 6 7 8 9 10 HIGH

6. Healthy thoughts

_____

_____

Certainty of beliefs   LOW 1 2 3 4 5 6 7 8 9 10 HIGH

7. Unhealthy reactions

_____

_____

8. Healthy reactions

_____

_____

9. Mindfulness and acceptance skills I have practiced

_____

_____

10. Visualizations I have used

_____

_____

11. Alternative skills I can use

_____

_____

12. Cognitive behavioral exercises I used to manage anxiety

_____

_____

13. Costs and benefits of my anxieties

_____

_____

14. Goal for managing my anxiety

_____

_____

Handout 2.7: Weekly Anxiety Record

Check off the practices you used this week and explain each checked item below.

_____ Mindfulness practices
_____ Challenging negative thoughts and cognitive distortions
_____ Thought logs
_____ Visualizations
_____ Cognitive defusion
_____ Eradicating the ANTS
_____ Experimental technique
_____ Downward arrow technique
_____ The "What if?" technique
_____ The feared fantasy technique
_____ Analysis of pros and cons/costs vs. benefits
_____ Flooding
_____ Gradual exposure
_____ Systematic desensitization
_____ Metaphors I have used to alleviate stress
_____ Using books and worksheets

In the space below, explain each checked item.

_____

_____

_____

_____

_____

Recommended Resources

Books for Clinicians and Clients

The Anxiety & Phobia Workbook
Edmund J. Bourne

When Panic Attacks: The New, Drug-Free Anxiety Therapy That Can Change Your Life
David D. Burns

How to Control Your Anxiety Before It Controls You
Albert Ellis

Get Out of Your Mind & Into Your Life: The New Acceptance & Commitment Therapy
Steven C. Hayes

Helping Your Shy and Socially Anxious Client: A Social Fitness Training Protocol Using CBT
Lynne Henderson

Mindfulness for Beginners: Reclaiming the Present Moment—and Your Life
Jon Kabat-Zinn

Thoughts and Feelings: Taking Control of Your Moods and Your Life
Matthew McKay, Martha Davis, and Patrick Fanning

Self-Help That Works: Resources to Improve Emotional Health and Strengthen Relationships
John C. Norcross, Linda F. Campbell, John M. Grohol, John W. Santrock, Florin Selagea, and Robert Sommer

The Mindful Way Through Anxiety: Break Free From Chronic Worry and Reclaim Your Life
Susan M. Orsillo and Lizabeth Roemer

Links

Anxiety and Depression Association of America
http://www.adaa.org

Beck Institute for Cognitive Behavior Therapy
"CBT Resources"
http://www.beckinstitute.org/what-is-cognitive-behavioral-therapy/

Belmont Wellness: Emotional Wellness for Positive Living

http://belmontwellness.com

(David Burns's logs)

http://sarahjourney.webs.com/index.html

Feeling Good: The Website of David D. Burns, MD

"Therapist's Toolkit"

http://feelinggood.com/resources-for-therapists/therapists-toolkit/

GET.gg Therapy Resources

"Cognitive Behaviour Therapy Self-Help Resources"

http://www.getselfhelp.co.uk/freedownloads2.htm

Kim's Counseling Corner

"Therapeutic & Self-Help Worksheets"

http://www.kimscounselingcorner.com/resources/therapy-and-self
-help-worksheets/

The Linehan Institute: Behavioral Tech

(Marsha Linehan's DBT site)

"Tools for Clinicians"

http://behavioraltech.org/resources/tools_clinicians.cfm

Mindfulness-Based Cognitive Therapy

http://mbct.com

Psych Central

"Anxiety: An Introduction to Anxiety Disorders" by John M. Grohol

http://psychcentral.com/disorders/anxiety/

"Using Mindfulness to Treat Anxiety Disorders" by George Hofmann

http://psychcentral.com/blog/archives/2013/01/28/using-mindful
ness-to-treat-anxiety-disorders/

Therapist Aid

"Worksheets"

http://www.therapistaid.com/therapy-worksheets/none/none

CHAPTER THREE

The Depression Solution
Beating the Blues

Depression and mood issues, along with anxiety, account for most of the material found in self-help and treatment workbooks for practitioners, affecting an estimated 19 million American adults each year. According to the Centers for Disease Control and Prevention, about 1 in 11 people have feelings of hopelessness and sadness that could justify a diagnosis of depression. Depression is a mood disorder that strikes people in all walks of life, of all ages, and at all socioeconomic levels in our society, making it one of the most common reasons that people seek counseling.

Due to its prevalence, depression is often considered to be the common cold of mental disorders. Clinical depression is a mental illness that can be costly and debilitating by adversely affecting the course and outcome of common chronic conditions such as arthritis, asthma, cardiovascular disease, and diabetes. It also contributes to increased work absenteeism, short-term disability, and decreased productivity. However, it is important to keep in mind that some depressive reactions are normal, such as in the event of the death of a family member or close friend. This is known as a reactive depression, and it does not necessarily trigger a long-standing impairment. Furthermore, many people use the term *depression* loosely to describe anything from getting up on the wrong side of the bed to thoughts of suicide. Regardless of whether the symptoms are life-crippling or more like a low-grade gnawing, there are some common treatment methods that can help your clients master their moods.

Much work has been done not just in the treatment of depression, but also in the prevention of it by way of life-skills training. For example, Yale professor Susan Nolen-Hoeksema (2004) found that women tend to have a more ruminative style, leading to depression, than men. Her research supports her thesis that females in particular tend to dwell on their problems rather than the possible solutions to their problems. With this realization, she spearheaded a school intervention program to teach adolescent girls (who are prone to rumination) emotion-regulation skills to help them handle their moods.

Martin Seligman, the father of Positive Psychology, spearheaded a depression-prevention project in schools in the Philadelphia area. In his book *The Optimistic Child* (2007), he details this successful program, which provided optimism-skills training. The children who received the skills training scored significantly higher in optimism and lower in depression in later years than the children who did not participate in the depression-prevention program. This shows that skills of optimism can be taught, a fact that can support clinicians' enthusiasm for providing clients with life-skills training to treat their depression.

The preventative life-skills research studies by Seligman and Nolen-Hoeksema are both examples of how psychoeducation is key in the prevention and treatment of depression. The psychoeducational components of Cognitive Behavior Therapy (CBT) and the third-wave approaches have provided a wealth of treatment strategies for treating depression. Thus, there is no shortage of interventions, and this chapter will condense the vast array of approaches by highlighting some of the most compelling and widely used solution-oriented treatment ideas.

The most popular model of treatment intervention is CBT. The effectiveness of CBT, founded by Dr. Aaron Beck in the 1960s, is well documented, and it is the most widely accepted approach to the treatment of depression around the world. A decade earlier, Albert Ellis laid the groundwork with his Rational Emotive Behavior Therapy (REBT) model, which Beck elaborated on, emphasizing the role of thoughts in creating feelings. The next section will help you educate your clients about CBT and on how they can change their thoughts to change their lives.

Treatment Tips

In starting treatment for almost any disorder, psychoeducational mini-lessons that introduce the rationale for using various treatment strategies and approaches are always helpful. In the case of depression, which is the focus of so much attention in clinical settings as well as in self-help books, CBT is a good place to start, as it is the most widely researched and applied treatment approach for depression. Following the first mini-lesson, which teaches clients the basics of CBT, I have outlined some essential CBT tips for structuring your session most effectively, followed by some treatment activities and exercises.

☑ *Mini-Lesson: CBT Basics*

Although Albert Ellis and Aaron Beck provided the foundation for CBT with the idea that disturbing feelings are caused by often-automatic disturbing thoughts, the roots of cognitive therapy go back to early philosophers like Epictetus in the first century AD:

People are not disturbed by things, but by the view they take of them.

It's not what happens to you, but how you react to it that matters.

A century ago, Einstein also realized that new ways of thinking are needed to supplant the ways of thinking that initially created our problems.

We cannot solve our problems with the same thinking we used when we created them.

Many clients come to counseling wanting to change how they feel and have no clue that changing their thoughts is the key. I always give my clients a mini-lesson on the importance of separating thoughts from feelings. Teaching your clients how thoughts are based on negative perceptions, and conveying that only by changing these thoughts and perceptions will feelings of depression subside, is best accomplished through using examples. I personally illustrate the cognitive model by using the case of one of my very first clients, a 17-year-old who ran in front of a car after her boyfriend broke up with her. This was back in the late 1970s, and a witness of the incident called the police. Luckily, my client was unharmed, and she was brought in a police car to the mental health clinic where I worked at the time.

Using an example like this one to teach my clients CBT concepts, I then use handouts such as "The ABC Depression Log" (Handout 3.2), which employs Albert Ellis's ABC model for REBT. However, I do not show them the handout at first, because they will think they already know the lesson, although many people don't think of it on their own. So, before showing them the handout, I tell my clients that I'm going to teach them the psychological ABCs. I draw *A*, *B*, and *C* on a piece of paper. After telling them the story of this client, I tell them (and write down on my paper) that *A* stands for *Activating Event* or *Adversity*, in this case the boyfriend breaking up with the client. I then write down on the paper that *C* stands for *Consequences*—the feelings (devastation) and the behavior (running in front of a car). I then ask my clients if *A* caused *C*—that is, did my client's boyfriend's breaking up with her cause her to run in front of a car? Most often, they think this is true. I then ask them what letter is between *A* and *C*, and of course they say *B*. I ask them what they think the *B* stands for—the thing that really made the young woman run in front of a car. They often say *behavior*, and I point out that behavior is under *Consequences*. My clients are then often blank as to what the word could be, even if I tell them it doesn't have to start with *B*. When I tell them that it was her *beliefs*—her thoughts, her perceptions—they are often surprised they didn't think of it, which is precisely the point. I tell them that our thoughts are often so automatic we're not even aware of them. We think that situations, rather than how we think and how we process them, cause our feelings and behaviors.

After going over this example, I show clients "My Daily Thought Log" (Handout 3.3). I instruct them to use the ABC model as a prototype for dissecting their own thoughts, feelings, and consequences. I also briefly introduce the *D* and the *E* columns, which stand for *Disputing* and the *Effects* of more rational thought, which is all described on the handout example. Many times I have my clients use this ABC log for homework between sessions, asking them to complete at least one or two entries each week to bring in to the next session so we can go over them together.

I show my clients that when people think irrational thoughts and make unhealthy conclusions, they feel upset and depressed. Healthy thinking is the key to feeling good.

In the weeks after introducing the topic of cognitive therapy, I continue to provide new skill-building worksheets, such as "Depression- and Anxiety- Producing Thought Habits" (Handout 3.4), at opportune times. A similar handout has already been provided in Chapter 2, on anxiety, but since depression and anxiety often go hand in hand and the illogical distortions are the same for both areas, I have included a similar handout for identifying distortions in both sections.

As you can see, CBT is an active approach that emphasizes self-help practice between sessions. Handouts, worksheets, and diary logs provide just some of the opportunities for work between sessions. Bibliotherapy, which constitutes recommending reading to clients, is also quite effective. One of the best self-help books is David Burns's *Feeling Good Handbook* (1999). I have supplied some other excellent bibliotherapy resources in the "Recommended Resources" section at the end of this chapter.

All these resources offer a great foundation for the practice of other CBT techniques between sessions. CBT encourages active self-help homework that involves practicing new skills and experimenting with challenging beliefs in the outside world. The following are CBT techniques that are quite effective in helping clients, both in session and also as they serve as their own best therapist between sessions.

☑ CBT Tip: Use CBT Diaries, Logs, and Skill-Building Worksheets

As already emphasized, the CBT approach makes heavy use of psychoeducational material. Mood diaries, thought and mood logs, worksheets, and handouts that help clients recognize and challenge irrational thoughts offer many opportunities to learn new CBT skills and apply them. Only by using self-help logs and worksheets will clients really be able to identify and tackle their irrational core beliefs at the root of their depression.

One of the most effective logs for depression is David Burns's Daily Mood Log (Burns, 1999; a link is included in the "Recommended Resources" section at the end of this chapter). It is laid out in four parts and serves as a good representation of the important elements in any CBT log:

1. Identifying the upsetting event.
2. Identifying the negative feelings.
3. A triple-column technique, in which the individual records an automatic thought (rating his or her degree of belief in that thought on a scale of 0 to 11), the type of cognitive distortion or thinking error inherent in that thought (chosen from a list of common cognitive errors), and the more rational thought that is substituted (rating the degree of belief on a scale of 0 to 100).
4. Outcome: After going through the other steps, the individual rerates his or her degree of belief on a scale of 0 to 100, deciding whether he or she feels not at all better, somewhat better, quite a bit better, or a lot better.

"Translating Irrational Thinking Into Rational Thinking" (Handout 3.7) is another example of a skill-building sheet that I use with clients. These types of worksheets make it very easy for clients to learn the basics of the CBT model.

☑ CBT Tip: Homework, Homework, Homework

Assign homework at the end of the session, and review it at the beginning of the next session.

The real effectiveness of CBT is often what happens outside therapy sessions. Therefore, when your clients come in with their worksheets and logs, it is important to start the session off by reviewing them with your client. If they are expected to do homework but it is not reviewed, it is less likely that they will take their homework seriously. By reviewing what they have done outside the session, you can help them correct any misunderstandings and clarify concepts that might be confusing to them.

☑ CBT Tip: Do a Mood Check
at the Start of Each Session

Judith Beck regards performing a mood check to be one of the most important elements of the beginning of each therapeutic interview, along with the review of the homework done between sessions. An informal, verbal mood check—that is, asking your clients how they are feeling—suffices in many cases. If feelings of depression are strong, then a more formal inventory like the Beck Depression Inventory is indicated. This widely used inventory consists of 21 multiple-choice questions to measure the severity of depression. Although it has gone though some revisions over the years since Beck formulated it in 1961, it has become widely accepted in the medical field as an acceptable instrument for measuring mood. Beck's Anxiety Inventory is also widely used to measure anxiety in a survey fashion.

In measuring and evaluating depression, Burns's Brief Mood Survey for Depression is also a handy form to have clients fill out before each session.

☑ CBT Tip: Use Bibliotherapy in Your Treatment
of Depression

Knowing which books to recommend for various client issues will ensure that your clients will be able to work at getting better between sessions, through education and skill practice contained in self-help materials. Self-help materials and therapy are a good combination. I keep a lending library for my clients, from which they can borrow some of my favorite self-help books to reinforce ideas we have discussed in session. Some of my favorites are included in the "Recommended Resources" list at the end of this chapter.

If your client is reading a self-help book you recommended between sessions, remember to follow up on how the reading went. Ask them if and how the reading has helped them. As with handouts, take the opportunity to clarify and expand on certain points in the book, clearing up any misconceptions.

☑ *CBT Tip: Help Clients With Goal Setting*

For the solution-oriented therapist, helping clients decide on goals for within and between therapy sessions is crucial for keeping treatment on track. Judith and Aaron Beck, as well as David Burns, rely heavily on goal setting at the beginning of the session. This ensures that therapist and client share the same goals for treatment. Starting each session by discussing goals for the session complements your review of the homework at the beginning of the session. The client and therapist also need to agree on methods to reach the goals, whether they be role-playing, filling out CBT logs, creating a cost-versus-benefits analysis, or tackling the depression scale each week before the session. This helps the client define the problem with the help of the therapist, and then implement a game plan for change.

Between-session assignments needs to be realistic, and at times they may require tweaking. Sometimes the client or the therapist misjudges how ready the client is to tackle a particular task. For example, after a role play, it is not unusual for my clients to feel ready to approach someone to have a much-needed discussion, only to find out that in the real world they are too intimidated. One particular client and I spent two sessions role-playing a difficult workplace situation. He was planning to go to his boss to express some problems he was having with coworkers in the department. He wanted to clear the air and figure out a solution so they could all work better together. I role-played the boss while the client played himself, then we reversed roles, and then we returned to our original roles. Even though we practiced a lot and planned to have him approach his boss the next week, he came back claiming that he was just not ready to try it in real life. We then revised our goals, breaking them down into more manageable steps. For example, the client felt more confident about approaching the boss about a less-threatening topic. He ended up changing his behaviors with his coworkers after getting more clarity on the workplace situation, so he ended up benefitting from the role play, but he never did actually have that discussion about them with his boss.

☑ CBT Tip: Ask for Feedback

Judith Beck emphasizes the importance of asking for feedback at the end of the session. I personally have been struck by how important asking for feedback has been, because sometimes the answers are quite surprising. My client's impression of a session and my impression occasionally are quite different. Feedback allows for clarification of misunderstandings and provides an opportunity to sum up the main points in the session. I often ask my clients to sum up what they have learned, because what I think they have learned and what they have actually learned are not always the same.

For example, in one session I told my client at the beginning of the session that I was going to be away for the next month on an extended vacation. When I asked her for feedback at the end of the session, she replied that she really didn't remember what we talked about because she was thinking about how she was too dependent on me and worried about her ability to handle not having sessions for a few weeks. She claimed that during the session she had started thinking that the transference and dependency were too much and that it was just wrong, causing her to feel ashamed, and she started thinking that maybe she would not continue therapy. She was having a whole internal dialogue, and unless I had asked for feedback, I would not have known. We ended up scheduling another session that week, since this was obviously an important topic to explore, and we both did not feel comfortable waiting for our next weekly session.

After that session, I began leaving more time at the end of sessions with this particular client to get feedback, and many times this has been beneficial to clear up misperceptions and unexpected reactions.

☑ CBT Technique: Coping Cards

Coping cards are an effective and widely used technique developed by Judith Beck at the Beck Institute for Cognitive Behavior Therapy. Coping cards are small note cards—perfect for your back pocket—that offer reminders throughout your day of positive thoughts that can help your clients cope.

There are different variations of coping card. Some are affirmations that clients can look at for support; others are reminders of skills clients can use when they feel depressed. Some are two sided, with one side containing a negative thought and the other side combatting that thought with a more rational alternative. I use them often with my clients to remind them of important points they need to remember in times of depression. Some of my clients have put clear contact paper over the cards and use a binder ring to hold them together, color coding the cards by type (for example, affirmations on blue cards and irrational versus rational thinking on pink cards). Below are some examples:

Coping Card Example 1:
Practical Coping Strategies for Stressful Times

When I am upset, I will:
- Read my coping cards
- Take a short walk
- Call a friend
- Journal
- Watch a taped show
- Do my needlework
- Read excerpts from my depression workbook

Coping Card Example 2: Irrational Thoughts on One Side, Alternative Rational Response on the Other, Including Type of Cognitive Distortion

Coping Card Side #1	Coping Card Side #2
I will never will be happy.	That is an example of fortune telling and all-or-nothing thinking. I am learning new skills and my happiness will be up to me.

Coping Card Example #3: Affirmations and Coping Self-Statements

I am a good person.

I am worthy of love.

I am proud of the way I keep trying to grow.

It's okay to make mistakes—it means I am human.

☑ *CBT Technique: Labeling Cognitive Distortions*

The hallmark of CBT is the labeling of types of cognitive distortion. This helps to make the irrational way of thinking more objective, enabling clients to understand the type of illogical reasoning underneath their irrational thinking. "Depression- and Anxiety- Producing Thought Habits" (Handout 3.4) and "My Mood Log" (Handout 3.6) are both excellent handouts for introducing the concept of labeling and teaching about the types of cognitive distortion. Handouts that identify cognitive distortions are also found in many cognitive therapy workbooks as well as in many mood logs, such as David Burns's popular Daily Mood Log. Examples of cognitive distortions are "shoulding," fortune telling, minimizing, personalizing, and black-and-white thinking. In my office, I keep a cognitive distortion list on hand to use when the discussion focuses on irrational thoughts. This handy list allows me to encourage my clients to identify the types of cognitive distortion they are experiencing.

☑ *CBT Technique: Getting to the Core Beliefs*

Core beliefs are one's fundamental assumptions about oneself, and in the case of depression, the core beliefs are faulty ones. Core irrational beliefs such as "I'm a loser" and "I'm a failure" are the breeding ground for many depressing interpretations of everyday events. The idea is that only by uncovering core irrational beliefs can people really change and improve their mood.

Judith Beck and other CBT notables stress the importance of using techniques to zero in on a client's basic beliefs. There are various ways to get to your clients to do this. A few of them are described next.

DIG DEEPER

Have your client imagine that a shovel is digging deeper and deeper until it reaches the root of the problem. This visualization will help your clients explore what is underneath a disturbing thought. Encourage your clients to keep digging deeper, until they hit bottom at their core belief. I use this image often with clients, and it helps them identify their core beliefs, which we then dispute together using a cognitive distortions sheet such as Handout 3.4.

This is an example of digging deeper to the core beliefs:

"I hope they like me"
"It would be terrible if they didn't like me."
"It would be terrible to make a mistake."
"They even think they are better than me."
"They *are* better than me."
"I'm a loser."

PEEL AN ONION

Another visualization is that of an onion. Have your clients imagine peeling off the layers to identify their core beliefs. In therapy, we can help our clients peel the layers of their defenses and their irrational thoughts to get to the core of their thinking.

THE DOWNWARD ARROW TECHNIQUE

One very popular technique used by David Burns to get to the core of irrational beliefs is the vertical or downward arrow technique, previously described in Chapter 2. In this technique, the therapist asks a client the same question each time the client mentions an irrational thought, getting to the bottom of their perceptions.

For example, I used this technique with a client who found many faults with the way she looked:

Client:	**Therapist:**
"I hate my nose and my hair— they make me so unattractive."	

                                    "If this were true, what would that
                                    mean to you?"

↓

"No one will find me attractive"

                                    "If this were true, what would that
                                    mean to you?"

↓

"I'll be alone the rest of my life."

                                    "If this were true, what would that
                                    mean to you?"

↓

"No one likes me."

                                    "If this were true, what would that
                                    mean to you?"

↓

Core belief: "I'm a total loser."

When my client and I got to her core belief, we spent less time focusing on her hair and nose and more time on her basic sense of low self-worth. Instead of reassuring her that her hair and nose were perfectly fine and trying to get her to accept them, I helped her to focus on her core beliefs underlying those critical thoughts. By identifying the core beliefs with the help of the vertical arrow technique, we chipped away at her absolute and distorted self-view, which stemmed from negative messages from childhood that she now regarded as fact. It is these main beliefs that need to be challenged so that the lens through which our clients look at the world will be clearer. Once you identify core beliefs with your clients, these beliefs can serve as a focus in their coping cards and thought logs, which will further help them to dislodge their fundamentally faulty views.

☑ CBT Technique: Shame-Attacking Exercises
Albert Ellis originally made this exercise popular, and it is still a popular CBT intervention. For clients struggling with anxiety and depression,

exaggerating a certain fear and acting on it can be empowering. For example, if your depressed clients is having a string of bad hair days and is unhappy with the way that she looks, a shame-attacking exercise might be to go up to strangers in a grocery line, for example, and say, "Wow, am I having a bad hair day!" Basically, by exaggerating her negative feelings about herself, she is pointing attention to her hair. This is a good exercise for clients who have body dysmorphic issues but are healthy enough to address them in this manner. It encourages them to have a sense of humor about their physical imperfections and not take themselves so seriously.

☑ *Behavioral Activation Strategies: Activity Monitoring and Activity Scheduling*

CBT therapists focus on the importance of *behavioral activation* techniques in the treatment of depression.

The term *behavioral activation* originated with behaviorist Charles Ferster (1973). This technique uses operant conditioning in the adoption of new behavioral habits to replace old avoidance habits. Clients create a hierarchy of reinforcing activities, in order of desirability or difficulty, using a token economy as reinforcement. For example, the more difficult an item is on the hierarchy, the bigger the reward. An example of an item on the hierarchy is calling three friends who have been out of touch. An example of a reinforcement is going to a movie you have wanted to see.

An important study on behavioral activation by Jacobson and colleagues (1996) found that for depressed people, writing out and structuring daily activities based on goals and values as a replacement for avoidant behaviors was just as effective as CBT psychotherapy. In this study, behavioral activation was found to be just as effective as CBT in helping clients with depression. Further studies showed that behavioral activation methods were even superior to medication alone in treating moderate to severe depression.

Behavioral activation comprises two parts: activity monitoring and activity scheduling. *Activity monitoring* helps clients recognize how they schedule their time. Clients are given a form to fill out describing what they do in a given day at every half hour or hour. The goal is to have your clients review how they spend their time so as to determine if they are spending too much time on one thing, such as playing video games or watching TV, instead of other activities they want to do, such as connecting with friends and family members.

Based on activity monitoring, the therapist and client then make an *activity schedule* using a hierarchy of goals, accompanied by reinforcements for completing the items on the hierarchy. It provides the tools and structure for making clients' time more productive in the pursuit of their goals.

Judith Beck emphasizes the importance of activity scheduling for depressed clients. Since depression leads to withdrawal from activities, helping clients reengage with activities in a structured way is crucial in helping them to be more active and engaged in life. Beck uses an activity chart that basically consists of a blank calendar with hourly intervals for clients to schedule activities. The idea is that when you write your activities down, you are more likely to complete them. These logs are then reviewed during the next session. David Burns (1999) also uses this method in his Daily Activity Schedule handout.

I have included a "Weekly Goal-Setting Inventory: Hierarchy of Activities" (Handout 3.5) in the "Handouts" section of this chapter to help you use the behavioral activation method with interested clients.

☑ CBT Technique: Cost/Benefit Analysis

In a cost/benefit analysis, clients write the *costs* or disadvantages of a depressing thought and then the *benefits* or advantages of hanging on to that thought. So, for example, my client who avoided going to parties listed as a benefit that he did not have to risk being rejected and feeling awkward, but the cost was that he felt lonely and isolated from others. After he listed more items on both sides, I asked him to choose percentages for both columns to indicate the strength of his reasoning, with those percentages equaling 100%. Thus, the Costs column got 35% and the Benefits column got 65%. It is not unusual for the Benefits side to win out, since after all, people are coming to therapy to make positive changes. When I brought my client's attention to the relative strength of the benefits, he became convinced that he should go to the party, and he was more confident in his decision than he likely would have been if he had not done this exercise.

☑ CBT Technique: The Acceptance Paradox

This CBT technique involves seeing the truth in self-criticism and individual shortcomings, and exaggerating them to make the shortcomings seem worse. Once your clients feel that they don't have to defend themselves and that they can accept their imperfections, to the point of exaggerating them, they have made a big step toward self-acceptance. An example, a client might say, "I really am a flawed human being who has made many, many mistakes. That's just me! I am a pro at making mistakes!"

For clients who are plagued with guilt and self-recrimination, this is one of my favorite techniques. When clients fundamentally believe they are at fault and are guilty for acting in ways that they now regret and are ashamed of, causing them to feel depressed and hopeless because they can't change the past, the acceptance paradox can provide much comfort. Instead of gearing therapy toward trying to get clients not to feel as guilty, just focusing on helping them to accept that they made errors and that they really didn't do such a great job at handling situations in the past can actually be freeing. Making the point that they have become wiser and can make different choices now is sometimes the best we can do. Basically, we are giving our clients permission to be human and flawed, and helping them to make peace with the fact that they are imperfect and a work in progress.

☑ Therapeutic Demonstration: Just One Negative Thought

Demonstrations can be quite effective to make important therapeutic points in both individual and group settings. Specifically, demonstrations can be very effective in helping clients to learn important concepts useful in combating depression. One of my favorites (which I often use as a visualization with individual clients) shows the power of one negative thought. I put one drop of food coloring into a clear glass of water, and everyone watches as the dye disperses and the water slowly changes color. I then ask my clients to imagine dropping many drops of food coloring—representing the many irrational, negative thoughts we often entertain during the day—into the water. I ask them to imagine the muddiness that results when toxic thoughts are mixed together. This illustrates the power of negative thoughts. This demonstration can also show, conversely, the power of even one positive thought and how it can color your world more positively!

☑ *Therapeutic Demonstration: It's Always Right Side Up!*

Give a round coffee filter to your clients. Have them write a negative thought on the bottom of it, and on the side facing up respond to that negative thought with a more positive one. Then have your clients stand up and hold the filter, bottom (negative) side up. When they let go, they will invariably see that the filter turns over and lands positive side up! This is a great group activity, as it makes an impact when many people simultaneously let go and watch everyone's filter turn right side up. The lesson is that positive thinking wins every time!

☑ *Therapeutic Demonstration: Our Perceptions Are Our Filter*

Using the coffee filter visual, I discuss with my clients the metaphorical meaning of the filter. It can be used to represent how our perceptions filter how we perceive the world. Sometimes our filter doesn't allow us to perceive things accurately—we get only some information through our filter. Also, I use the filter to show that whenever anyone says something to us, we need to filter it and not personalize it so that we can stay protected. For example, someone's words could be very hurtful if we don't take into account that what people say often says more about them than it does about us.

☑ *Therapeutic Demonstration: Irrational Songs*

In a group situation, play short excerpts of irrational songs (for example, from iTunes or even YouTube) to demonstrate how we learn to think irrationally, and to drive home the point that only by challenging these irrational thoughts can we fight depression and anxiety.

Some of my favorites examples are:

"I Can't Stop Loving You," performed by Ray Charles
"You've Made Me So Very Happy," performed by Blood, Sweat &
    Tears
"There Goes My Everything," performed by Englebert Humperdinck
"You Make Me Feel Like a Natural Woman," performed by Aretha
    Franklin

Using these examples, make the point that no one can actually make you feel a certain way, and that by thinking more rationally you can take your power back. A lack of power is directly linked to depressive thinking. My clients love this music demonstration, and especially in group situations, playing a short excerpt from each song on my iPhone makes for a humorous and dynamic interchange.

☑ *Quick Mindfulness and Acceptance Practices*

Many of the third-wave approaches to treatment combine CBT techniques with mindfulness and acceptance practices. These approaches make liberal use of metaphors, visualizations, and acronyms to teach skills of acceptance and present-centeredness. These are a nice addition to your therapeutic toolbox, especially when you are working with particularly hard-to-treat clients who are resistant to change despite a good foundation of CBT principles.

Here are a few of my favorites:

Leaves floating on a stream. This is a visualization from Acceptance
    and Commitment Therapy (ACT) founder Steven Hayes, in which
    clients are instructed to imagine putting each of their negative
    thoughts and negative labels about themselves on a leaf (one for
    each thought), and then to watch those leaves float away and
    eventually disappear. Clients experience watching their thoughts
    rather than feeling stuck with them inside their head. One of my
    very treatment-resistant clients has found this visualization to be
    one of the most helpful things we have ever done in six years of

therapy, and she uses this often between session when she gets overwhelmed with feelings of depression and anxiety.

The Yellow Jeep. This is another visualization from Hayes, showing that when we resist our thoughts, we end up focusing on them more. In this activity, clients are asked to think of a yellow Jeep, and then to stop. It's hard to stop! Thus, traditional thought-stopping practices that used to be so popular in CBT have been determined to be ineffective, since you are fighting your thoughts rather than accepting them and detaching from them. This practice helps underscore to clients the importance of accepting some inevitable pain in their lives instead of spending all their effort resisting it.

Cognitive defusion. Another ACT practice (previously introduced in Chapter 2) is having clients learn skills to distance themselves from their thoughts so that they can stop being judgmental, by looking *at* their thoughts objectively rather than *from* them. They observe that they are thinking distressing thoughts, rather than thinking them without suspending judgment. For example, they might think, "I am having the thought that I am a loser" rather than "I am a loser."

☑ Helping Your Clients Get "Connected"

Depression leads to loneliness and loneliness leads to depression; subsequently, they feed on each other. Often people who report sadness and depression isolate themselves, whether from a lack of energy or fear of rejection or from just not knowing what to say or do. And this isolation leads to more depression.

One of the most important things that therapists can do is take an inventory of their clients' social connections and determine if their clients have at least one person in their lives around whom they can "be themselves" and with whom they can self-disclose.

Shawn Anchor, author of *The Happiness Advantage* (2010), spent years at Harvard studying the importance of job satisfaction, social connection, and support on the job. He found that productivity and job satisfaction were directly correlated with the degree of perceived social support.

He also cites a study, conducted with 1,600 Harvard students in 2007, that uncovered a strong correlation between social support and happiness. He says, "So if in the modern world we give up our social networks to work away from friends and follow celebrities on Twitter, we are trading off with our happiness and health."

In this day and age, the term *getting connected* often refers to using the latest wireless technology and social apps. Connecting through Internet groups such as Facebook certainly is one of the ways our clients stay connected with family and friends, but sometimes just the old-fashioned way of keeping connections is what people are missing in their lives.

The worse you feel, the harder it is to get "out there," and by feeling isolated, clients are more likely to feel sad and preoccupied with their own internal self-talk. This leads to further avoidance of social interactions. Helping clients to reconnect with the outside world is often an important focus in counseling and can be the subject of between-session assignments.

Therapists often make the error of focusing on the client's individual issues to the exclusion of helping them assess whether they are connected enough to sustain healthy relationships. I have also emphasized to my clients that joining a religious or interest-related group can help lessen their depression due to the social support that comes with belonging. At other times, just making the decision to open up to a trusted friend or relative can help clients feel less alone and depressed.

For example, a shy, depressed, 42-year-old school nurse felt anxious around her peers and lacked confidence in her ability to relate to just about anyone, including her husband and his family. She habitually declined invitations from school staff to go to happy hours, due to a discomfort of socializing outside of work and also due to a fear that her controlling husband would be angry if she didn't come right home. I encouraged her to make an effort to attend even one happy hour, not expecting to be part of the "in crowd" but just being there as an observer and making polite conversation. I emphasized the importance of getting social support in getting better and feeling less depressed.

To her surprise, she had a lot of laughs and fun at the happy hour, and eventually she became an organizer of happy hour activities. She started to make friendships with a few staff members outside of school and began setting better limits with her husband.

It is important to note that encouraging this client to connect more with others would not have worked if she hadn't been given the tools to become more assertive and identity her rights, all of which are addressed in Chapter 6.

A Toolkit of Metaphors for Treating Depression

Coffee filter. The coffee filter reminds clients of two of the demonstrations in the Treatment Tips section. The coffee filter reminds us that the positive side always wins, and also represents the importance of keeping in mind that our perceptions filter our reality and how we see the world.

Arrow shape. This arrow can be drawn on a note card, or it can be an arrow sticker or an arrow cut out of construction paper. In times of difficulty, your clients can remember to identify their core beliefs by using the downward arrow technique and digging deeper to uncover their core beliefs.

Coping cards. For the depressed client, putting a few coping cards in the depression toolkit will offer some perspective in times of low mood. In keeping with the metaphorical theme, you can have your clients draw or cut out from a magazine or download from the Internet a picture that represents to them a depression-busting image. One example would be a picture of a favorite flower that grows from the dirt and darkness to bloom beautifully in the sunlight.

Smiley face sticker. It is important to smile! Studies have shown that even the act of smiling can lighten mood.

Plastic leaf. This can be a trigger for remembering the ACT exercise "Leaves on a Stream," reminding your clients to look *at* their thoughts rather than *from* their thoughts.

Colored pencil or paintbrush. A reminder that our attitude colors our world.

Therapeutic Takeaways

☑ CBT techniques and resources offer many psychoeducational avenues for treating depression in and out of session.

☑ There are various forms of self-help diaries, mood logs, coping cards, tracking sheets, and skill-building worksheets to help clients learn skills to fight depression. Cognitive worksheets help clients identify faulty thought habits.

☑ CBT techniques such as the vertical arrow technique and shame-attacking exercises help clients combat depression.

☑ Behavioral activation techniques, comprising activity monitoring and activity scheduling, help clients become more proactive and reduce the effects of depression.

☑ Mindfulness and acceptance practices help clients become more present focused, less judgmental, and more accepting.

☑ The importance of social connectedness cannot be overemphasized in dealing with depressed individuals. Helping your depressed client connect with others is crucial to successful treatment.

Handouts

The following sample worksheets will help your clients develop skills to fight depression. The worksheets are all related to the lessons of this chapter. As a general guideline, handouts and assignments are given to your clients at the end of the session as homework, unless they are used in the session itself to illustrate points. Make sure you leave ample time to go over your expectations regarding the use of the selected handout.

When assignments are given out, it is important to follow up with your clients at the beginning of the next session by reviewing and discussing their homework with them. Going over the homework is an essential aspect of being a solution-oriented therapist.

Note: All handouts in the book are available for download on my website by following the link below: http://www.belmontwellness.com/ultimate-solution-handouts/

Handout 3.1: Common Myths About Depression

Myth 1: Depression is always a psychiatric disorder.

Depression is a state of low mood that forms a continuum from feelings of sadness to severe, life-crippling clinical depression. It may last for hours, days, or even years. The important thing to note is that depression is not necessarily a clinical issue. Some people use the term loosely to point to an underlying sense of moodiness that comes and goes, and at times might be part of someone's DNA.

Even though it may not meet the requirements for a psychiatric disorder from a clinical standpoint, depression is nonetheless a mood issue and often a reason for seeking professional help. It is also important to note that some depression is a normal reaction to life events, and again cannot be termed a disorder. Examples of inciting events include:

1. The breakup of a relationship
2. Death of a loved one
3. Loss of a job
4. Moving away from friends and family
5. Going through the holidays when loved ones are no longer able to be there due to death or distance

Sometimes depression is a side effect of drugs, postpartum blues, or coping with illness.

Myth 2: People who are depressed are weak and should be able to "snap out of it."

Depression is an illness, and thinking that people should snap out of it is like saying they should not have cancer or that they should not be hungry before mealtime.

Depression is not something to be ashamed of, and in fact, the more it is suppressed, the more it remains and grows, just like a tumor. Instead of defending against feelings of depression, it is healthy for people with depression to recognize those feelings, which will enable them to work toward getting the help they need.

Myth 3: Using medication for depression is a cop-out, and once you start, you will depend on it.

Clients often say that they want to beat depressive feelings themselves without help. Although there is nothing wrong with initially trying to use nonpharmaceutical methods, there are times that medication is desirable—and even necessary—in tackling low moods.

Medication alone is typically less effective than when it is used in conjunction with therapy. Taking medication because of a stressful life event does not mean a lifetime of dependency. It can be viewed as an aid during a time of recovery and healing.

I often use the metaphor of a microwave with clients. Medication is like using a microwave oven—you can defrost a chicken on the counter, but it will take a lot longer than if you defrost it in the microwave.

Myth 4: In most cases, depression is not curable.

Depression is generally curable, but the approach to treatment is not one-size-fits-all. Some people respond well to medication, while others respond well to a cognitive behavioral approach—without medication—to change their thoughts and their moods.

In the current psychotherapy environment, there are many treatment strategies that offer hope and healing to almost all types of depressive symptoms.

Myth 5: It's best to keep feelings of depression to yourself, because talking about it makes it worse.

Actually, depression is best helped when it is shared with others. Isolating yourself with feelings of depression often make it worse, and it festers. Many times, unhealthy depressive thoughts multiply and are exaggerated in the mind, and only by talking and sharing can they be processed.

Handout 3.2: The ABC Depression Log

A Adversity or Activating Event	B Depression-Causing Beliefs	C Consequences: Feelings	C Consequences: Behavioral Reactions	D Disputing Belief	E Effects of Disputing the Belief
Example: Boyfriend cheated on me	I am nothing without him. He ruined my life. He was the only one for me.	Devastated Depressed Angry Rejected	Withdrawn Hostile Overeating and drinking Short fuse with family and friends	He does not make me worthy; I am worthy no matter what. He has no power to ruin my life.	I am sad he was not trustworthy, and will be more careful to look at red flags when I am in another relationship.

Handout 3.3: My Daily Thought Log

	Irrational Thoughts	Certainty of Beliefs (%)	Types of Cognitive Distortion	Alternative Rational Thoughts	Certainty of Beliefs (%)	Action Plan and Goals
1						
2						
3						
4						
5						

Sample Types of Faulty-Thinking Habits

1. *CATASTROPHIZING.* You label things as horrible and awful instead of unfortunate or disappointing: *"This is HORRIBLE!"*
2. *FORTUNE TELLING.* You think you can predict the future: *"I'll never find anyone who will be interested in me. I'll be alone the rest of my life."*
3. *BLACK-AND-WHITE THINKING.* You make all-or-nothing assumptions: *"All men are bad."*
4. *PERSONALIZATION.* You blame yourself for things that are out of your control: *"I am to blame for my child's issues."*
5. *JUMPING TO CONCLUSIONS.* You make assumptions and regard them as fact: *"He told me he can't come to the party. I bet he just doesn't like me."*
6. *LABELING.* You label yourself and others instead of being specific. Instead of saying, *"I made a mistake,"* you label yourself a *"failure"* or a *"loser."*
7. *MAGNIFICATION.* You make mountains out of molehills: *"This is the worst day of my life."*
8. *MINIMIZATION.* You deny that things are an issue when they are: *"It's not a big deal"* (when it really is) or *"I don't care"* (when you really do).
9. *"SHOULDING."* You have a judgmental attitude toward yourself and others: *"He shouldn't be so upset about it"* or *"I should be smarter and thinner."*
10. *MAKING COMPARISONS.* You compare yourself to others: *"He is so much smarter than me."*
11. *MENTAL FILTER.* You focus on one negative detail and not the whole picture, discounting the positives: *"I am ugly because of my large nose."*

Handout 3.4: Depression- and Anxiety-Producing Thought Habits

Irrational Thoughts *Example:* "I am a loser and always will be."	Types of Cognitive Distortion "Labeling, fortune telling, all-or-nothing thinking"

Sample Types of Faulty-Thinking Habits

1. **CATASTROPHIZING.** You label things as horrible and awful instead of unfortunate or disappointing: *"This is HORRIBLE!"*
2. **FORTUNE TELLING.** You think you can predict the future: *"I'll never find anyone who will be interested in me. I'll be alone the rest of my life."*
3. **BLACK-AND-WHITE THINKING.** You make all-or-nothing assumptions: *"All men are bad."*
4. **PERSONALIZATION.** You blame yourself for things that are out of your control: *"I am to blame for my child's issues."*
5. **JUMPING TO CONCLUSIONS.** You make assumptions and regard them as fact: *"He told me he can't come to the party. I bet he just doesn't like me."*
6. **LABELING.** You label yourself and others instead of being specific. Instead of saying, *"I made a mistake,"* you label yourself a *"failure"* or a *"loser."*
7. **MAGNIFICATION.** You make mountains out of molehills: *"This is the worst day of my life."*
8. **MINIMIZATION.** You deny that things are an issue when they are: *"It's not a big deal"* (when it really is) or *"I don't care"* (when you really do).
9. **"SHOULDING."** You have a judgmental attitude toward yourself and others: *"He shouldn't be so upset about it"* or *"I should be smarter and thinner."*
10. **MAKING COMPARISONS.** You compare yourself to others: *"He is so much smarter than me."*
11. **MENTAL FILTER.** You focus on one negative detail and not the whole picture, discounting the positives: *"I am ugly because of my large nose."*

Handout 3.5: Weekly Goal-Setting Inventory: Hierarchy of Activities

Rank goals for the week in order of difficulty, 1 being the most difficult and 10 being the least, and indicate with a check mark which days you worked on each goal. To gain a sense of mastery, start with the least difficult first.

Hierarchy of Goals and Activities

	Most Challenging Goal	S	M	T	W	T	F	S	Progress Notes
1									
2									
3									
4									
5									
6									
7									
8									
10									
	Least Challenging Goal								

Handout 3.6: My Mood Log

Use the following log to track your mood and emotions, identifying the beliefs and behaviors that result.

Mood Analysis	
Negative Emotions	Positive Emotions
Strength of Negative Emotions 1 2 3 4 5 6 7 8 9 10 Low High	Strength of Positive Emotions 1 2 3 4 5 6 7 8 9 10 Low High
Identify Negative Beliefs	Challenge With Positive Beliefs
Cognitive Distortion	Challenge to the Cognitive Distortion
Certainty of Your Beliefs 1 2 3 4 5 6 7 8 9 10 Low High	Certainty of Your Beliefs 1 2 3 4 5 6 7 8 9 10 Low High
Unhealthy Behaviors	Healthy Behaviors
Cost/Benefit Analysis: Unhealthy Coping	Cost/Benefit Analysis: Healthy Coping
My Conclusions and Goals	

Handout 3.7: Translating Irrational Thinking Into Rational Thinking

In this handout, notice how unhealthy thinking can be translated into much healthier and more flexible thinking when you take away rigid, judgmental negative interpretations.

At the bottom of the list, use your own examples to be a positive emotional translator!

Irrational Thoughts	Rational Alternatives
I can't stand this!	This is disappointing.
It's TERRIBLE!	It's unfortunate.
I'm stupid.	I made a mistake.
I *need* him/her to do that.	I *would like* him/her to do that.
Things always go wrong.	I feel as if things often go wrong.
I always goof up.	I am learning from my mistakes.
Life should be fair.	I wish life were more fair.
I should have known.	I wish I had known.
I am a loser.	I am a person with low self esteem.

Now it's your turn to translate. Think of some of your irrational thoughts and translate them into more rational thoughts.

Irrational Thoughts	Rational Alternatives
_____	_____
_____	_____
_____	_____
_____	_____

Handout 3.8: Weekly Depression Log

Date(s): _____

1. Upsetting event:

_____

2. Emotional responses:

_____

3. Degree of depressed feeling: LOW 1 2 3 4 5 6 7 8 9 10 HIGH
4. Depression-producing thoughts:

_____

   Certainty of beliefs: LOW 1 2 3 4 5 6 7 8 9 10 HIGH
5. Depression-busting thoughts:

_____

   Certainty of beliefs: LOW 1 2 3 4 5 6 7 8 9 10 HIGH
6. Unhealthy reactions:

_____

7. Healthy reactions:

_____

8. CBT skills I have used to combat depression:

_____

9. Mindfulness and acceptance skills I have practiced:

_____

10. Alternative skills I can use:

_____

11. Costs and benefits of my depressive thinking:

_____

12. Action plan and goals for combatting depression:

_____

Recommended Resources

Self-Help Books

The Feeling Good Handbook
David D. Burns

Feeling Good: The New Mood Therapy
David D. Burns

Mind Over Mood: Change How You Feel by Changing the Way You Think
Dennis Greenberger and Christine A. Padesky

The Cognitive Behavioral Workbook for Depression: A Step-by-Step Program
William J. Knaus

Thoughts and Feelings: Taking Control of Your Moods and Your Life
Matthew McKay, Martha Davis, and Patrick Fanning

The Mindful Way Workbook: An 8-Week Program to Free Yourself From Depression and Emotional Distress
John Teasdale, Mark Williams, and Zindel Segal

The Mindful Way Through Depression: Freeing Yourself From Chronic Unhappiness
Mark Williams, John Teasdale, Zindel Segal, and Jon Kabat-Zinn

Clinician Books

Cognitive Therapy of Depression
Aaron T. Beck, A. John Rush, Brian E. Shaw, and Gary Emery

Cognitive Behavior Therapy: Basics and Beyond
Judith S. Beck

86 TIPS (Treatment Ideas & Practical Strategies) for the Therapeutic Toolbox
Judith A. Belmont

127 More Amazing Tips and Tools for the Therapeutic Toolbox
Judith A. Belmont

Rational Emotive Behavior Therapy: A Therapist's Guide
Albert Ellis and Debbie Joffe Ellis

Cognitive Therapy Techniques: A Practitioner's Guide
  Robert L. Leahy
Skills Training Manual for Treating Borderline Personality Disorder
  Marsha M. Linehan
The CBT Toolbox: A Workbook for Clients and Clinicians
  Jeff Riggenbach

Links

Beating the Blues: Cognitive Behavioural Therapy
  www.beatingtheblues.co.uk
Beck Institute for Cognitive Behavior Therapy
"Cognitive Therapy Rating Scale (CTRS)"
    http://www.beckinstitute.org/SiteData/docs/CTRS122011/3388
    12377f0513fe/CTRS%2012-2011_portrait.pdf
(Depression Inventories and Scales)
    http://www.beckinstitute.org/beck-inventory-and-scales/
"Burns Triple Column Technique"
    http://www.power2u.org/alternatives2013/downloads/Burns-Triple
    -Column-Technique.pdf
"Therapist's Toolkit"
(from David Burns)
    http://daviddburnsmd.files.wordpress.com/2014/01/aaa-tk-order
    -form-website-v-1-2014.pdf
National Institute of Mental Health
"Major Depression Among Adults"
    http://www.nimh.nih.gov/statistics/1mdd_adult.shtml
Psych Central
"Depression" by John M. Grohol
    psychcentral.com/disorders/depression
Psychology Tools
"Free Cognitive Behavioural Therapy (CBT) Worksheets and Self-Help
  Resources"
    http://www.psychologytools.org/download-therapy-worksheets.html

CHAPTER FOUR

The Anger Solution
Giving Up the Grudge

Our clients commonly have the misperception that anger is an emotion that is inherently bad. This accounts for why anger is such a problem for so many of them. When it is denied and suppressed for too long (just like stress), it usually ends up resulting in emotional struggles as well as contributing to major relationship problems. Whether anger leads to eruptions and outward conflict or an internal buildup that is expressed in less direct ways, it becomes toxic to our lives. Freud himself considered anger turned inward to be a major cause of depression.

Well over 2,000 years ago—long before the field of psychology was established—even Buddha has something to say about anger, which rings just as true now as it did then:

> *Holding on to anger is like grasping a hot coal with the intent of throwing it at someone else; you are the one who gets burned!*

Mark Twain also spoke on the dangers of festering anger:

> *Anger is an acid that can do more harm to the vessel in which it is stored than to anything on which it is poured.*

Medical studies have supported these analogies, concluding that true physical ailments and even premature death are linked to extreme forms of anger. One of the best-known and conclusive studies focused on the

Type A personality. In the 1950s, cardiologists Meyer Friedman and Ray Rosenman (1959) found that the chance of coronary disease doubles in men from the ages of 35 to 59 if they have a Type A personality. Type A characteristics are found in workaholics who are driven, impatient, and overly ambitious. Later, however, these researchers clarified that ambitious Type A personalities without the anger factor are actually not more prone to heart disease and other ailments than their less-driven Type B counterparts. It was determined that it is really the *hostility* factor combined with a Type A personality which makes people more prone to heart disease.

It is important to note, however, that anger is not necessarily bad if it is properly channeled and spurs on constructive action. Anger that spurs action constructively does not impair our health. Most of us can think of examples of clients or people we know who have made the world a better place because they channeled their anger into constructive action. For example, the organization Mothers Against Drunk Driving (MADD) was founded in 1980 by a mother of a 13-year-old who was killed by a drunk driver. This major societal movement, which supports, educates, and seeks legislative changes in regard to how drunk drivers are dealt with, was built on the outrage of personal injustice and serves as a shining example of how anger can lead to our improving our quality of life. The solution-oriented therapist has a unique opportunity to teach their clients about the tools and skills they need to manage their anger instead of carrying it and endangering their health and well-being. (Notice that *anger* is one letter short of *danger!*)

Help your clients uncover the cognitive distortions that lie beneath unhealthy, out-of-control anger. Often, at the peak of emotion, people are so blinded by anger that they are unaware that inflexible, faulty cognitive distortions are feeding it. They tend to blame someone else for making them feel so angry. They are unaware—especially in the moment —that they possess the ability to deescalate the rage that they feel when other people won't change or do what they want them to do. To help your clients identify common anger-producing cognitive distortions use Handout 4.6 ("Common Anger Cognitive Distortions"), based on the works of CBT notables like Beck and Burns. To explain each type of anger-producing cognitive distortion featured in the first treatment tip. I use the example of my client, Susan, a newly divorced mother of two who was prompted to come to counseling by her anger at her ex-husband and her difficulty accepting her new life as a divorced woman.

Susan came late to her second session, claiming that her ex-husband "made her late" as he wouldn't let her off the phone in her car. Referring to her ex-husband as a "jerk," she added, "and that's a fact!" Once we discussed the common cognitive distortions behind anger, she realized the absurdity of the labeling (stating an attribution as a fact), and only then could she lighten up about her ex-husband and stop being so immobilized by her anger. Months later, when she was again late to a session, she chuckled when she talked about the original incident, realizing that her "facts" were actually her gross misinterpretations. By stopping the irrational thoughts, she felt as if she got her life back.

In dealing with intense anger, as in dealing with many other common client symptoms such as anxiety and depression, a focus on cognitive distortions is quite helpful. Recognizing faulty thinking patterns is the first step to changing them. Using some of my handouts on cognitive distortions with Susan helped her to identify that she was using all-or-nothing thinking, labeling, and overgeneralization.

Treatment Tips

In my practice, I enjoy using a variety of tools that I can apply to a client's specific issues in response to anger. Some of them are activities that I assign for homework, such as reading handouts and filling our worksheets between sessions; and we do some of the worksheets together during session. I also use visualizations or metaphors to illustrate a certain point. The following treatment tips are among the most effective in my anger solution toolkit.

☑ CBT Technique: Identifying Common Anger-Producing Distortions

In this "Treatment Tips" section, using the example of my client, Susan, who was mentioned in the introduction, I will demonstrate the usefulness of identifying the type of cognitive distortion to calm down angry thoughts.

The following common anger-producing cognitive distortions were pointed out to Susan. She was able to reexamine her faulty habits of thinking and replaced these errors of thought with more healthy and manageable ways of thinking.

LABELING

Labeling is stating an interpretation about someone's character as a fact, often to the point of demonizing someone. Once clients demonize someone and think in terms of labels, their anger can easily turn to fury and in some cases leads to verbal and even to actual physical assault. Teaching your clients the perils of labeling will help them defuse the intense anger and demonization that prompted them to behave badly. In the case of my client, Susan, she learned to replace labels for her ex-husband with healthier terms:

Anger-Producing Distortions	Corrections of Cognitive Distortions
He is evil!	*He has a lot of problems and is very unhealthy.*
He's a jerk—and that's a fact!	*I am upset with him and think many things he has done are not right.*
He's psycho!	*I find his behavior very disturbing.*

THE "SHOULDS"

Shoulds and *musts* regarding how other people act are one of the greatest triggers of anger. Judging how others *should* act and what they *should* do erodes relationships and is the source of constant conflict. Help your clients to be a *should* detective. Use the image of a magnifying glass to remind them not to *should* on others! (Note: I purchase toy magnifying glasses in bulk online and give them to my clients to help them to be *thought detectives* and identify their *shoulds*.)

Anger-Producing Distortions	Corrections of Cognitive Distortions
He shouldn't be acting like that!	*I wish he didn't act that way.*
He should have known better.	*I wish he had known better.*
He shouldn't keep me on the phone when he knew I had an appointment.	*He did not make me stay on the phone—I allowed him to and gave him power over me.*

BLAMING

Blaming is one of the most common types of cognitive distortion, and one that can lead to unhealthy anger and rage. When your clients are stuck in blame, they surrender their power and give the power to the person they are mad at, making them more angry. By taking more responsibility for her own feelings instead of blaming her ex-husband for them, Susan was able to think in "victor" language and not "victim" language:

Anger-Producing Distortions	Corrections of Cognitive Distortions
He upset me.	*I am upset with him.*
He pushes my buttons!	*I am in charge of my buttons and it is up to me to not allow him to push them.*
He is the reason I am miserable.	*I feel miserable because of how I respond to him.*

BLOWING THINGS OUT OF PROPORTION

Assumptions that are perceived in absolute terms, rather than in flexible, rational terms, result in all-or-nothing thinking and blow things out of proportion. These cognitive distortions are immobilizing and lead to thinking that is rigid while at the same time grandiose. Susan learned to think in ways that are more specific and less overwhelming. She learned to avoid absolutes like "never" and "always":

Anger-Producing Distortions	Corrections of Cognitive Distortions
He NEVER appreciated my family!	*I was disappointed how he did not mix well with my family.*
He ruined my life!	*My life is not ruined—I am going through a rough time.*
He ALWAYS tries to get his way.	*He often tries to get what he wants without compromise.*

MIND READING

It is one thing to assume, and another to think you know why someone is doing something. Clients who practice mind reading often personalize what others are thinking and doing to slight them. Susan learned that her tendency to mind read limited her ability to see things objectively.

Anger-Producing Distortions	Corrections of Cognitive Distortions
He is trying to make life difficult for me.	*I will not speculate—I am not in his head.*
He is trying to make me feel guilty.	*No one can make me feel guilty except me. This is just my interpretation, not fact.*

FORTUNE TELLING

People who get angry often feel a sense of hopelessness and get to the point where they feel as if their anger is the "last straw." Fortune telling is like thinking you can predict the future. Susan's problems were made worse because she felt she could predict the future, and in her hopeless state, could not see light. Fortunately, she learned to challenge her predictions as fears and not facts:

Anger-Producing Distortions	Corrections of Cognitive Distortions
I'll never get over how he treated me!	*It will be hard for me to get over that.*
He'll never learn!	*He is very resistant to change.*
I will never find someone else.	*It is hard to imagine finding someone to love again.*

The resources in the handout section provide opportunities for your clients to practice labeling and changing their cognitive distortions. "Common Anger-Producing Cognitive Distortions" (Handout 4.7) and "Anger-Producing Thoughts and Healthier Alternatives" (Handouts 4.3 and 4.4) will help your clients identify their anger-producing distortions.

☑ CBT Exercises: Anger Logs and Diaries

Using my client Susan as an example, we have seen how various types of cognitive distortions cause a great deal of mental distress. In learning how to correct those distortions, Susan was able to move on with her life and react to her ex-husband's consistently challenging behavior from a place of empowerment and not weakness.

Once you help your clients to identity their faulty distortions, providing them with an anger log (Handout 4.5) will help them track their thoughts, emotions, and behaviors related to their feelings of anger.

To let your clients know that you take their homework seriously, I recommend spending at least the first 5 minutes of a session going over homework; this also allows you to gauge their progress in handling their anger. Cognitive behavior therapy (CBT) and third-wave treatments all emphasize the importance of encouraging clients to use logs in mastering feelings associated with anxiety, depression, and anger. Once your clients start to identify the thoughts and events that trigger their anger, they are likely to gain a more rational perspective and replace their irrational thoughts with more rational ones.

Possible components of an anger log include:

Triggering thoughts

Triggered behavior

Type of cognitive distortion

SUDS rating (subjective units of distress, 0–100)

Anger-producing alternative thought

Alternative feelings and behaviors based on healthier thinking

In many cases, the effectiveness of using these handouts is contingent on how we as therapists follow up with our clients and review their worksheets and logs. Allotting time at the beginning of the session to review homework sends the message to clients that homework is essential to their progress. It helps them process the work they have done in session and reinforces its value, and it can also help to clarify for them what areas they need to work on in session. Handout 4.8 ("My Weekly Anger Summary") also gives your clients the opportunity to practice their skills in managing anger between sessions.

☑ Mini-Lesson: Anger as Pain

For all types of disturbing symptoms, psychoeducation is key in helping clients develop more insight and the ability to change. My clients are often very surprised to learn that anger is frequently an expression of pain, and this shift in perspective opens their hearts to be able to give up some of their judgmental anger, giving way to heal with compassion.

People get angry and feel life is unfair when things don't turn out the way they want, or when others don't act or think the way they want them to. When anger is viewed as an expression of pain, treatment focuses on efforts to manage the pain and the painful triggering thoughts. Being aware of the anger–pain connection will shift attention from grudges and bitterness to healing from the pain and loss that is really at the root of clients' anger. Getting to core beliefs has been a cornerstone of CBT, and one of the most powerful core beliefs of angry clients is that they are powerless because life did not work out the way they had hoped it would or the way they thought they deserved it to.

Michelle was a client who was outraged by the behavior of two coworkers who seemed to be marginalizing and undermining her in various situations at work. She came to counseling all fired up because these two coworkers, many years her junior and much less experienced, had ended up getting chosen for a special project that she herself had requested. She was angry also at the way her boss seemed to favor them, and found herself vacillating between ignoring them and having tense and terse exchanges with them. In counseling she realized that her sense of indignation about the unfairness of it all triggered feelings of being in middle school, where she had been marginalized by the "popular" group. She recalled that she had even been sent to the principal's office because of her negative behavior resulting from her sense of injustice. Twenty-five years later, the memories still hurt. Upon further exploration, she admitted that growing up she had felt as if her brother was favored over her, and the memories still hurt even though her mother was long deceased.

Michelle and I worked on helping her to forgive her parents and schoolmates for not being as kind as she would have liked, and in the process I went over with her "The Five Stages of Grieving and Healing" (Handout 7.5). She grieved the loss of the chance to have a better relationship with her parents as well as the loss of the expectation that her childhood and her work situation would be as fair and satisfying as she would have liked them to be. She worked to forgive people in her past that did not treat her as well as she would have liked, and stopped focusing on how her coworkers should be different, becoming more accepting of them for who they were. Once she let go of the need to "make things right," she was able to trade her focus on what "should" be with a focus on appreciating the many positive things in her life. In accepting that life was not always going to be fair, she began to embrace her imperfect world, and in all areas of her life began to shift from anger to acceptance. (It's important to emphasize to your clients that acceptance is not merely feeling defeated and resigned. Rather, it means adopting a nonjudgmental attitude toward what cannot be changed and detaching from its power to define you.)

I offered Michelle sheets like "Common Anger-Producing Cognitive Distortions" (Handout 4.6), and she began to identify her tendency to "should," blame, and blow things out of proportion. "My Anger-Producing Cognitive Distortions Log" (Handout 4.7) provided the opportunity for her to identify her own unique distortions and write out more rational alternatives. The worksheet on "Anger-Producing Thoughts and Healthier Alternatives" (Handout 4.4) offered her additional practice opportunities to identify irrational thoughts and she was better able to replace them with more rational alternatives.

Now that Michelle's distorted thoughts had been addressed, the next stage of therapy focused on developing better communication skills in times of anger. She learned that acceptance of life's unfairness did not mean caving in to it and lashing out at others.

☑ Mini Lesson: The Difference Between Anger (a Feeling) and Aggression (a Behavior)

First, Michelle needed a primary education on the basic types of communication: *assertive*, *nonassertive*, and *aggressive*. Two of my favorite handouts for teaching clients the difference are "The Three Types of Communication" (Handout 6.2) and "Comparing the Three Types of Communication" (Handout 6.3). With handouts like these as a basis, Michelle learned that when she was angry, she did not have to become aggressive. She had always confused the two, as many of our clients do. I followed up the psychoeducational handouts with skill-building worksheets for identifying the anger-producing internal self-talk that led to her aggressive reactions (Handouts 4.3 and 4.4, "Anger-Producing Thoughts and Healthier Alternatives").

Over time, I used additional communication skills worksheets, such as "Turn *You* Statements Into *I* Statements" (Handout 6.4) and "Aggressive Behavior: Reasons, Payoffs, and Consequences" (Handout 6.5), which further educated her on the reasons behind her aggressive behavior and helped her to differentiate an aggressive communication style from her angry feelings, which she could choose to express assertively. Worksheets like these provided Michelle with a good foundation for learning tactful communication. "Common Myths About Anger" (Handout 4.1) also helped her to correct some of her misperceptions concerning anger.

The case of Michelle represents many lessons we can learn about solution-oriented treatment. We need a lot of tools in our toolbox from various life-skills areas to tailor treatment to our clients' unique needs. Insight into their pain is the first step—but we need to put at their fingertips practical resources for learning new ways of thinking and behaving. Showing clients *how* to make changes and giving them the means to do so will help them find solutions to almost any problem they face.

For Michelle, what started as a focus on her outrage at her coworkers became a lesson in healing from her troubled way of thinking, paving the way for the building of calmer ways of coping with improved communication skills.

☑ Experiential Activity: Use Role Play to Transform Aggression Into Assertion

The above-mentioned communication handouts from Chapter 6 can be used in carrying out role-playing with clients to help them express their anger assertively, which is often essential to addressing anger constructively. I have spent a good deal of time role-playing with clients to help them learn ways to handle challenging situations with tact. This will be discussed further in Chapter 6, but communicating assertively and not aggressively is so crucial to healthy interpersonal relationships that it bears mentioning in this chapter on anger.

Role-play is one of my favorite techniques to use with clients, and the benefits in preparing them for real-life situations are enormous. Not only does role play help clients to practice skills and prepare for real-life situations, but it also helps them to develop an assertive mindset and healthy way of thinking. In essence, our clients' own self-talk becomes more assertive—meaning that they learn to talk more assertively to themselves! After all, healthy self-talk is the foundation of healthy communication with others.

Through role-play, clients learn to anticipate issues that might come up and practice managing them tactfully. Many times I reverse roles with my clients, having them take the roles of people in their life who pose challenges to their assertiveness, and I can then model healthy communication skills. After they get some ideas of alternate responses, we switch roles so they can try out their new assertiveness skills.

Make liberal use of role play to help teach clients to replace aggressive communication with assertive communication. Even though role-play is not "real life" and is carried out in the comfort of my office, I have been struck by how nervous, upset, and angry people get just acting out their real-life situations. Role-play has by far been one of the best activities I have found for helping clients learn to handle their anger appropriately and use their anger constructively rather than destructively.

☑ CBT Technique: Cost/Benefit Analysis

Cost/benefit analysis is a very useful technique for helping your clients evaluate the pros and cons of their anger. There are some payoffs of anger, as there are for any other emotion or behavior, even if they are not obvious. Label one side of a piece of paper the "Benefits" column and the other side the "Costs" column, and the reinforcers for carrying out certain undesirable behaviors become clearer. Now, taking another piece of paper, make columns for the costs and benefits of alternative behaviors. After all lists are completed, have clients rate how strongly they feel about their beliefs, with the percentages on each paper equaling 100% combined. Usually the "Costs" column of the undesired behavior and the "Benefits" column of the alternative behavior are given much more weight, which may help motivate clients to make positive changes.

A cost/benefit analysis can be done both in session and between sessions at regular intervals if symptoms persist. It is advisable to do this exercise together in session the first time so that you can help your clients process the activity.

☑ CBT Technique: Use Anger Reducing Coping Cards

In many of the chapters in this book, coping cards are recommended because they are so powerful in helping to keep clients on track through focusing on healthy coping strategies. This could not be more important than in the case of anger. Clients need healthy reminders, available at a moment's notice, to help them remain calm and stable. Encourage your clients to carry rational self-statements in their pocket, purse, backpack, and so forth so that they will always be accessible. Having coping cards available is especially important for grounding when clients are anticipating situations that might trigger anger. Examples of anger-reducing coping cards are "Remember to visualize a stop sign," "I won't give anyone power over my feelings—I am in control," and "Be careful of my 'shoulds' about him. It's not that he 'shouldn't' act that way—it's that I wish he did not." Self-statements can serve as mantras to keep mentally focused and disciplined—and putting them on a coping card can help remind clients to keep calm when anger is aroused.

Writing appropriate phrases on coping cards, on Post-it notes, or on a computer screen can help clients stay focused when their anger is triggered. For a group activity, brainstorm phrases and healthy reminders to write on coping cards. Compile a list of coping self-statements on a board or flip chart, and then give out note cards so that group members can write out the coping statements from the list that they might find helpful when they're angry. Here are some mantras that my clients have found helpful when their anger is triggered:

"Just stick to the facts, not interpretations."
"No one makes me feel any way—I allow them."
"No one has power over me unless I give it to them."
"Count to 10 before responding."
"If you can't fight it, and can't flee it, then flow with it. "
"Anger is one letter short of DANGER."

Can you and your clients think of other statements to add to the list?

☑ Activity: Turn Anger Into Goals

As previously emphasized, anger can be a good motivator for constructive action. After all, anger is a catalyst for action, and healthy actions can result from strong feelings if they are channeled into goals for making things better. Using Handout 4.2 ("Turning Anger Into Goals"), clients can get practice turning an angry thought into a goal for constructive action. For example, "She is so unfair" can be transformed into a goal like "Since she does not treat me fairly, I have even more reason to work on my assertiveness and stand up for my rights." I often emphasize to my clients that having challenging people in their lives gives them an opportunity to work on their assertiveness issues. I encourage them to be thankful for having someone in their life with whom they can react against—look at how much they can learn about themselves! This attitude helps clients reframe their anger into something positive.

☑ *Humor Strategies: Focusing on using humor to heal*

One thing about anger is that all too often it makes people quickly lose all sense of humor. This is why clinicians need to help clients appreciate and enact the power of humor, because a sense of humor puts things in perspective and helps defuse anger.

One of the ways to help clients use humor as a means of deescalating anger is to model that use of humor. This does not mean laughing at your client, of course! The humorous approach of paradoxical intention can at times help defuse anger and help clients gain a more rational perspective. In paradoxical intention, the therapist intentionally uses a gross exaggeration to make a point about the client's unhealthy stance, to the point of absurdity. For example, if a client is furious about having to put up with her ex-husband because of the kids, you can suggest to her that she can imagine herself as a martyr or goddess for putting up with him, or imagine herself receiving a big medal. A bit of humorous exaggeration can offer perspective and goes a long way toward defusing anger.

☑ *Visualizations: Helping clients use images to heal*

Visualizations can be a powerful means of helping clients to control their anger. They help reduce emotional distress by creating some sense of distance with the use of images, and they can help clients shift from focusing on their emotional pain to regarding the intense emotion as an experience to learn from. Visualization helps clients focus their imagination on healthy images that can serve as a guide and a reminder to engage in healthy coping, which comes in handy during times of emotional duress.

THE TIP-OF-THE-ICEBERG VISUALIZATION

This is a very effective visualization. Draw the image of an iceberg on a piece of paper with an individual client. Where the tip of the iceberg is protruding out of the water, write "angry outburst" or "angry feeling." Then, beneath the water line, write out all the thoughts that resulted in the angry outburst, such as:

"He shouldn't act that way!"

"I'm wasting my life."

"After all I have ever done for her—and she is so ungrateful!"

"I never thought my life would turn out like this!"

This helps clients become more aware of what is really going on behind their angry feelings and words.

This short activity can also be done in group settings using a flip chart or whiteboard. Here, as in individual sessions, it is quite effective in helping clients visualize what messages they are telling themselves under the surface that result in their angry feelings, thoughts, and behaviors.

THE ANGER THERMOMETER VISUALIZATION

The anger thermometer is great for helping clients of any age, including children, to visualize their anger. Find or create a picture of a thermometer that goes from 1 to 10. The numbers 1 through 10 represent gradations of feelings of anger, ranging from mild annoyance to rage. Once your clients identify where they are on the thermometer, you can brainstorm ways to lower the temperature from "seeing red." Visualizations such as these are useful in helping your clients get control over their anger and appreciating the intensity. I have included a link to an anger thermometer in the resources section at the end of this chapter.

SIGNS AND STOPLIGHTS VISUALIZATIONS

When clients figuratively *see red*, helping them to actually visualize the red image of a stop sign might help them control their impulses and *STOP* and think. Clients can conjure up internalized images from everyday life in times of emotional arousal and help keep their emotions in check—or at least their behaviors.

I also have my clients imagine a stoplight. When they are angry, they are seeing red. This is when it's time to STOP and not react, so as not to lose control. Next, I have them think of a yellow light and CALM DOWN and use caution with how they react and what they say. When they are calm, then they can "think green" and give themselves a "go" to express themselves.

Whether your client uses the simpler visualization of a stop sign or the more complex visualization of a traffic light, the benefits of stopping and thinking before reacting will likely save them from numerous interpersonal conflicts just by the bite of the tongue with the help of these two common visualizations!

You can brainstorm with your clients what other traffic signs can serve as warnings to them. For example, a yield sign can help clients remember that it is important to compromise in times of anger. A detour sign reminds them that sometimes we need to be patient and some paths are not so direct and straightforward.

Visualizations which involve objects that are common in everyday life have had a strong appeal with my clients, and they have remarked that when they drive in their daily lives, they are constantly triggered by the lessons of these common visualizations represented by traffic signs and lights, helping to keep them "in check."

THE FINGER TRAP VISUALIZATION

The classic finger trap is a perfect metaphor for showing how angry exchanges, as in an argument, trap both of the people who are trying to prove they are right. I buy them in bulk from an online discounter and often give them to my clients to help them remember not to get stuck in the "trap." By holding on to anger and the need to be right, you end up stuck in a relationship trap as well as trapped in negative thinking.

☑ *Mindfulness and Acceptance Strategies:* *Observing and Describing*

There are times when cognitive treatment alone is not enough to help a client shift away from old, rigid habits of thinking. For particularly treatment-resistant clients, the addition of mindfulness to your anger management toolbox is crucial. In the early 1990s, Dialectical Behavior Therapy (DBT) founder Marsha Linehan introduced Eastern mindfulness practices into the traditional cognitive approach in her management of treatment-resistant clients, such as suicidal clients, including the highly impulsive borderline personality population. Her thought was that for these populations, something else was needed in addition to

CBT techniques (Dimeff & Linehan, 2001). In fact, even the word *dialectic* (meaning "opposite") points to the integration of two seemingly opposed treatment strategies: acceptance-based practice and change-based practice.

In the acceptance-based module of her approach, Linehan's theory focuses on the importance of core mindfulness skills, allowing clients to deal with intense emotion by using mindfulness techniques. Throughout the book, various acceptance-based techniques are offered. In this section, I will use the example of the practices of observing and describing, which relate to the treatment of anger.

Acceptance strategies emphasize a non-judgmental stance in observing and describing what you sense. Observing and describing are examples of core mindfulness skills that help emotionally distressed clients develop a non-evaluative stance when they are emotionally triggered. *Observing* is the act of taking in sights, sounds, smells, and thoughts without labeling or judging. *Describing* is the act of putting words to those sensations without interpreting them. By using practices such as these, a client will become more likely to take a mindful, non-judgmental stance instead of giving in to extreme emotions.

Observing is geared toward quieting and calming the mind, which is just what angry clients need to cope with their emotional arousal. By practicing being non-judgmental, clients will develop the skills to calm their mind, and these skills will already be established when times come up that are upsetting. Linehan recommends the daily practice of just sitting and allowing oneself to observe one's surroundings, without judgment. Thus, instead of thinking, "I don't like this color yellow in the room," clients suspend judgment and just observe the walls without making any interpretation. The act of stepping back and observing will help clients develop a sensitivity of all five senses—hearing, smell, touch, sight, and sound. Instruct your clients to put aside times to be still and observe all sensations from their five senses, letting the mental chatter and commentary come and go. This practice has been described as using a *Teflon mind* where painful and anger-producing thoughts and feelings do not *stick*.

The focus on describing with non-judgmental awareness, as with a

Teflon mind, will help your clients put into words what they observe. For example, if one looks at the yellow paint on the walls, the description would be "The walls are painted yellow"—not that the walls are dingy or in need of repainting, or that the color is too dull or bright. Describing involves simply recording what is observed, putting it into words in the absence of judgment.

When I teach the act of describing to my clients, I scrunch my face up and ask them to *mindfully describe* what they see. Often the responses range from "angry" to "disapproving" to "upset." I teach my clients that these are just interpretations, and that mindfulness techniques stick to the observable facts and is quite different from idiosyncratic perceptions. I teach them that it is not that there is anything wrong with having interpretations in our lives as long as we know they are interpretations and do not regard them as facts. It is just that it is all too common when our clients are angry that they fuse their interpretations with facts and are not aware that they are being judgmental, leading to significant emotional distress. I teach them that if they were to mindfully describe my expression, they might say that I had "pursed lips," "a furrowed brow," "a tightened face," and so forth instead of assumptions about my feelings and mood.

By learning the technique of describing, clients will increase their ability to de-escalate their emotions in times of anger.

A Toolkit of Metaphors for Treating Anger

Use these metaphorical objects to remind your clients of the skills they need to control their *anger* so it won't end up getting them in *danger*! Some of the objects in this section were mentioned earlier in the chapter. These are examples of items that I keep in my office that are useful in helping clients visualize concepts related to anger and other mental health issues.

> **Small Teflon mini-spatula.** This spatula will help your clients learn to cope with anger by keeping a "Teflon mind" where thoughts are released easily and not letting their angry thoughts "stick."

The finger trap. Finger traps are inexpensive metaphorical objects that can make quite an impact and represent various lessons about conflict. This carnival toy represents what happens during an angry exchange—both people in an argument get stuck in the trap! Only by letting go instead of pulling (and proving you are right) can you get out of the trap and be set free.

Timer. A toy hourglass timer reminds clients to give themselves a time-out and not react impulsively when they are very angry. It helps to remind them to take some time before expressing anger. Similar to the common practice of counting to 10 before responding in times of anger, a 2- or 3-minute toy timer is a great reminder for helping your clients manage their anger. It can also help them set limits on how much time they will give themselves to stew in anger. Once the hourglass runs out, they need to turn it over again if they choose to continue stewing.

Toy thermometer. This reminds clients of the anger thermometer visualization, helping them observe their anger and equate its level of intensity to degrees on a thermometer.

Traffic signs. Whether the traffic lights, stop signs, and yield signs are downloaded pictures from the Internet, simply drawn on a card, or purchased from an online toy or hobby distributor, these can be useful in helping clients manage their anger. These images were explained in the visualization activities section under "Treatment Tips." In essence, imagining a big stop sign can help clients curb their impulse to speak in anger. The yellow light on a stoplight reminds them to use caution in times of anger, and the green light is the image they can visualize when they are calm enough to express themselves assertively. The yield sign is a reminder to compromise in dealing even with difficult people.

Feather. Feathers can be purchased from hobby stores. Just like feathers that are let out of a pillow, words spoken in anger cannot be taken back once they are back "out there."

Can you and your clients think of any more metaphorical objects to help them control their anger? This is a great group activity!

Therapeutic Takeaways

☑ Educate your clients that anger is a normal emotion. Just as we need stress, we need feelings of anger to motivate us and help us make changes. The problem arises when anger gets out of control, leading to out-of-control behavior.

☑ Help your clients identify the common cognitive distortions that interfere with handling anger effectively, such as labeling, fortune telling, "shoulding," blaming, blowing things out of proportion, and mind reading.

☑ There is an important distinction between feeling angry and being aggressive. Anger is a feeling and is acceptable, aggressive behavior is not.

☑ Mindfulness strategies can complement CBT strategies in helping clients calm down their angry emotions.

☑ There are many techniques for helping your clients manage their anger, such as various visualization exercises, including those involving stop sign, stoplight, anger thermometer, and tip-of-the-iceberg visualizations.

☑ An anger log and other anger worksheets will remind your client of important tips for managing their anger.

Handouts

The following worksheets will help your clients manage their anger. They are all related to the lessons of this chapter. As a general guideline, handouts and assignments are given to your clients at the end of the session as homework, unless they are used in the session itself to illustrate points. Make sure you leave ample time to go over your expectations regarding the use of the selected handouts.

When assignments are given out, it is important to follow up with your clients at the beginning of the next session by reviewing and discussing their homework with them. Going over the homework is an essential aspect of being a solution-oriented therapist.

Note: All handouts in the book are available for download on my website by following the link below: http://www.belmontwellness.com/ultimate-solution-handouts/

Handout 4.1: Common Myths About Anger

*Myth 1: Anger is an unhealthy and negative emotion
and should be avoided.*

Anger is actually a normal emotion that is needed for living a complete and well-functioning life. Anger is part of living that helps us react to situations in an appropriate way.

For example, if someone insults you or calls you names, anger is an appropriate feelings because your rights were being violated. Anger helps you stand up for what you believe in and is often the impetus for healthy change. Rosa Parks, Mahatma Gandhi, and Martin Luther King Jr. were effective because they did not accept the status-quo notion that people of their race were second-class citizens. Rather, they were angry enough to bring about positive changes in the world. However, they were not aggressive.

Myth 2: Anger means that behavior is aggressive.

Anger and aggression are often confused, and this remains the main reason why anger is so often seen in a negative light. The distinction between them is very important. Anger is a *feeling*, and is part of a normal gamut of human emotions, while aggression is a *behavior*.

Except when it is necessary to maintain personal safety or the safety of others in response to a physical attack or threat, aggressive behavior is not appropriate. By definition, aggressive behavior is disrespectful, meant to demean someone, change others, tell others what to do, and get your own way.

Myth 3: Anger is uncontrollable.

If we can exercise self-control, we can control how our anger is expressed. Anger doesn't have to be like an uncapped bottle of soda pop that fizzles and explodes when it is shaken and uncapped. Anger can actually be quite controllable. The more skills you have to manage and handle intense emotions, the more you will be able to handle anger rather than letting it all out. Anger becomes destructive when it is uncontrolled, which usually entails trying to control another person. Interestingly enough, the more you try control others, the more out of control you become!

Myth 4: Other people can make us angry.

When you think that other people can make you angry, you give the power to them; you believe they are making you feel like your anger is out of control. However, if you think assertively and accept that no one has the power to make you angry unless you give it to them, you'll find that your anger is much more under control.

Just as no one can change the neurons in your brain, no one can change your emotions and your perceptions. Your triggers may be external, but your emotions and reactions belong to you alone. If everyone had this understanding, it would eliminate many arguments and conflicts, which often arise when people feel as if they are victims, that they are not in control of themselves, and that there is no way out.

Myth 5: Anger is more common in men than in women.

Men and women both get angry, but men often express it in more overt and louder ways: i.e. aggressively. So it is not that women don't also get angry, but they have been socialized to express it differently. Through conditioning in our society, women are often encouraged to suppress their anger and be "ladylike" and "not make waves," whereas anger expressed by men is more acceptable and even rewarded in our society.

When men are angry, their reactions tend to be more physical and violent, whereas women are less likely to get physical with their anger. After anger is released, women tend to hold on to their anger longer than men—perhaps because women limit how their anger is expressed.

Myth 6: People tend to get more angry with age.

To the contrary; with age comes wisdom and perspective, and most people's anger and aggressive behavior decline with age. Individuals who tended to be aggressive as parents tend to be much more mellow with their grandchildren and their own children as they age. The urge to control others is lessened.

Handout 4.2: Turning Anger Into Goals

Use anger to motivate you to make your life better, instead of letting it stop you from pursuing your goals. Turn the following thoughts around to transform your anger into motivation for pursuing what is really important to you in your life.

Angry Thought   **Goal**

He is so unfair!   I will work to express myself and stand up for my rights.

I have the worst luck!   I am motivated to work harder to increase my odds.

I can't stand it!   I will develop skills to tolerate what I don't like.

Now it's your turn. Write down your angry thoughts and turn them into goals.

Angry Thought   **Goal**

_____   _____

_____   _____

_____   _____

_____   _____

_____   _____

_____   _____

Handout 4.3: Anger-Producing Thoughts and Healthier Alternatives

The table below will help you generate examples of anger-producing thoughts as well as healthier alternatives. Our thoughts—not other people—create our anger! To use as a model, Handout 4.4 offers examples of common anger practices, thoughts, and healthier alternatives.

Anger-Producing Thoughts	Healthier Alternatives

Handout 4.4: Anger-Producing Thoughts and Healthier Alternatives, Completed

The table below shows examples of anger-producing thoughts as well as healthier alternatives. Our thoughts—not other people—create our anger!

Anger-Producing Thoughts	Healthier Alternatives
I hate him!	I really do not like him.
She makes me nuts!	I get unstable in my reactions.
It's awful!	It's very disappointing.
She has no right!	I don't like how she behaves.
This shouldn't be happening!	I wish this weren't happening.
He ruined my life!	I am upset with him.
He has to stop doing that!	I will ask him to stop doing that.
He better not get away with it!	I hope he faces consequences.

Handout 4.5: My Anger Log

To fill in this log, think of a situation in which you felt that your anger got out of control.

Triggering Event	Triggering Thoughts	Behavioral Response	Types of Cognitive Distortion	Rate SUDS (Subjective Units of Distress) from 1–100	Anger-Reducing Alternative Thought	Alternative Behaviors

Handout 4.6: Common Anger-Producing Cognitive Distortions Sample

Anger-Producing Distortions	Corrections of Cognitive Distortions
Labeling	
"He is evil!"	"He has a lot of problems and is very unhealthy."
"What a jerk—and that's a fact!"	"I am upset with him and think many things he has done are not right."
"He's the devil!"	"I find his behavior very disturbing."
"Shoulding"	
"He shouldn't be acting like that!"	"I wish he didn't act that way."
"They should appreciate all I've done for them."	"They don't seem to realize what I'm try to do for them."
"He shouldn't tell me how I should feel!"	"I'm disappointed that he feels he has a right to tell me what to do and how to feel."
Blaming	
"He upset me."	"I am upset with him."
"He pushes my buttons."	"I am in charge of my buttons and shouldn't allow him to push them."
"She makes me so mad!"	"I was angry when she said that."
Blowing Things out of Proportion	
"This is horrible!"	"This is unfortunate."
"He is ruining the vacation."	"It has been challenging to be on the vacation with him."
Mind Reading	
"He is trying to provoke me!"	"It seems like he says things to try to make me lose my temper."
"He *hates* me!"	"He doesn't seem to like me, or at least like what I said."
Fortune Telling	
"He'll never change."	"I hope he can change his behaviors."
"I will never get over this!"	"I'll have to work hard to get over this one."

Handout 4.7: My Anger-Producing Cognitive Distortions Log

Using Handout 4.6 as a sample, identify your own anger-producing distoritions and h ealthier responses.

Anger-Producing Distortions	Corrections of Cognitive Distortions
Labeling	
"Shoulding"	
Blaming	
Blowing Things out of Proportion	
Fortune Telling	
Mind Reading	

Labeling. Labeling is stating an interpretation about someone's character as a fact, often to the point of demonizing someone.

"Shoulding." "Shoulds" and "musts" regarding how other people act are one of the greatest sources of anger.

Blaming. Blaming is when you feel like a victim, and believe that others are at fault for your feelings and reactions.

Blowing things out of proportion. This involves making rigid assumptions that show all-or-nothing thinking, or phrasing perceptions in absolutes rather than in flexible, rational terms.

Mind reading. Mind reading is when you make assumptions that people are doing something to you on purpose, or jump to conclusions, treating attributions as fact rather than opinion.

Fortune telling. To believe that nothing will change and that "things will always be like this" is a form of predicting the future.

Handout 4.8: My Weekly Anger Summary

Date(s): _____

1. Anger-provoking events

_____

2. Emotional responses

_____

3. SUDS (subjective units of distress) rating

                         LOW 1 2 3 4 5 6 7 8 9 10 HIGH

4. Unhealthy thoughts

_____

        Certainty of your beliefs   LOW 1 2 3 4 5 6 7 8 9 10 HIGH

5. Healthy thoughts

_____

        Certainty of your beliefs   LOW 1 2 3 4 5 6 7 8 9 10 HIGH

6. Unhealthy reactions

_____

7. Healthy reactions

_____

8. Mindfulness and acceptance skills I have practiced

_____

9. Rational thinking skills I have practiced

_____

10. Coping cards I have used

_____

11. Costs and benefits of my anger

_____

12. My plan for managing anger

_____

Recommended Resources

Self-Help Books

Prisoners of Hate: The Cognitive Basis of Anger, Hostility, and Violence
Aaron T. Beck

Act on Life Not on Anger: The New Acceptance & Commitment Therapy Guide to Problem Anger
Georg H. Eifert, Matthew McKay, and John P. Forsyth

How to Control Your Anger Before it Controls You
Albert Ellis and Raymond Chip-Tafrate

The Cognitive Behavioral Workbook for Depression: A Step-by_Step Program
William J. Knaus

The Anger Control Workbook: Simple, Innovative Techniques for Managing Anger and Developing Healthier Ways of Relating
Matthew McKay and Peter D. Rogers

Clinician Books

ACT Made Simple: An Easy-to-Read Primer on Acceptance and Commitment Therapy
Russ Harris and Steven C. Hayes

Cognitive Therapy Techniques: A Practitioner's Guide
Robert L. Leahy

Motivational Interviewing: Helping People Change
William R. Miller and Stephen Rollnick

Changing for Good: A Revolutionary Six-Stage Program for Overcoming Bad Habits and Moving Your Life Positively Forward
James O. Prochaska, John C. Norcross, and Carlo C. DiClemente

Links

HelpGuide.org
"Anger Management"
http://www.helpguide.org/mental/anger_management_control_tips_techniques.htm
"Kassinove & Tafrate's Anger Thermometer"
http://www.counsellingconnection.com/wp-content/uploads/2008/01/anger-thermometer.gif

CHAPTER FIVE

The Procrastination Solution
Helping Your Clients Implement Good Habits

Regardless of the clinical nature of a client's reasons for seeking treatment, a common by-product of our clients' symptoms is putting off important tasks, known as procrastination. Procrastination is the avoidance of performing a task that needs to be completed, choosing easier and more desirable activities instead. After all, much of our clients' energy is already depleted through dealing with their own emotional and relationship issues, and disciplining themselves requires a lot of work, effort, and motivation, which sometimes seems nowhere to be found.

Although few of our clients seek treatment for procrastination itself, issues related to procrastination usually end up being a main focus of treatment. The more depressed, anxious, and stressed our clients are, the less likely it is that they will have the discipline to implement positive new habits.

It is not uncommon for our clients to say that they will try to lose weight, stop smoking, and exercise more when they feel less stressed, but those feelings of shame and discomfort—especially if they are overweight and sedentary—keep furthering their stresses so that they never seem to be able to break the cycle.

Thus, many of the things that people put off changing are practices that give them some pleasure and comfort, even if the habits are bad for them, such as smoking, drinking, emotional eating, avoiding exercise, and so forth. Some activities such as watching TV, Internet surfing, and video games are diversions from working on emotional issues. Both the pleasure of these habits and avoidance of the hard work of improving oneself leave our clients less motivated to work on changing ingrained habits. It's difficult for them to surrender old, comfortable habits until they are feeling better, but it is precisely the act of procrastination that prevents them from getting better. It becomes a catch-22. The fallout from this stalemate is the guilt and low self-esteem that ultimately interferes with all aspects of their life, whether at work, school, or home.

Helping clients develop the motivation and commitment to implement strategies that will change their lives is an important focus of treatment. It's one thing to want to change and another to have the organized and proactive mindset to make the change. The solution-oriented therapist provides skills and strategies to help clients *get going* in order to eliminate bad habits and implement healthier ones so that the guilt of inactivity does not exacerbate other issues that brought the client to counseling.

Therapists traditionally believe that an important part of their job is to help clients clarify their values and treatment objectives and prioritize their goals. Taking it a step further by helping clients create an action plan and teaching them skills that will allow them to enact changes is a key to the success of solution-oriented treatment.

After all, our clients know they need to change; the problem is that many times they do not have the right tools or know *how* to change. Not knowing how to get motivated, practice, and organize time effectively leads people to procrastination. The solution-oriented therapist who provides clients with strategies to prioritize goals and helps them create action plans by breaking larger goals into smaller, more manageable goals will be most effective in moving them from talk to action. As with most client problems, psychoeducation is often the first step. It is easier to change if you are rooted in a foundation of knowledge. Educating our clients about the myths of procrastination (Handout 5.1) is a good first step in helping them make behavioral steps to change.

Although clients might see themselves as "lazy" due to their procrastination and use this explanation as a way to beat themselves up (which increases their depression and anxiety), we can help our clients normalize their procrastination by exploring the common, underlying themes of procrastination. Some of these are fear of failure, perfectionism, "shoulding" on themselves, and feeling forced rather than feeling like they have a choice.

Fifty-three-year-old Jessica, for instance, just didn't want to make the "wrong" choice. The house that she and her husband had bought five years back needed much work, and although they had the money to fix the house up, she felt immobilized to make decisions. Her husband worked long hours at the company he had founded, and when they bought the house, Jessica had agreed to be in charge of renovations. However, except for the things that had needed to get done, such as getting a new hot water heater, nothing had been done even after five years. Jessica's husband was becoming increasingly frustrated because the house was in disrepair, even though it was functional. In exploring the issues that caused her procrastination, Jessica claimed that she was overwhelmed by the choices and did not want to make a decision she would regret. She felt she already had many regrets in her life, and she claimed that she could not bear having one more.

We will now focus on some of the solutions to the prevalent problem of procrastination.

Treatment Tips

☑ *Self-Help Worksheets, Tests and Surveys:*
Practicing Skills Between Sessions

David Burns's Procrastination Test (1999, p. 171) provides a 10-item survey of common attributes that lead people to procrastination. After completing the survey, clients rate how much they agree with each statement on a scale of 1 to 4. For example, one of the items is "I sometimes procrastinate because I'm afraid of failure."

Once underlying emotional barriers are identified, they can become the focus of treatment. For example, in the face of perfectionism, David Burns offers a two-column technique that he refers to as "Perfectionism vs. the Healthy Pursuit of Excellence" (1999, p. 176). Through the use of this technique, irrational fears related to perfectionism are answered in healthier and more logical ways, just as cognitive distortions are answered with more rational alternatives.

Using the example of Jessica, this is an example of how she would fill out this self-help sheet.

Perfectionism	Pursuit of Excellence
I am motivated by fear of making the wrong choice.	*I am motivated by enthusiasm for being creative and creating a beautiful place.*

This technique is similar to another of Burns's techniques— performing a cost/benefit analysis.

☑ CBT Technique: Cost/Benefit Analysis

The cost/benefit analysis is a mainstay of Cognitive Behavior Therapy (CBT). To use this technique with your clients in session, together write down the pros and cons of procrastination in a particular situation, the pros in one column and the cons in the other. Below is an example of a list that might be created by a client who puts off organizing her cluttered house.

Benefits	Costs
It is more fun to do fun stuff.	*My house is cluttered and I cannot find things.*
It's messy again anyway.	*It will always be messy if I never organize.*
I won't give in to my spouse's nagging.	*It is causing stress in our relationship.*
I don't want the time pressure.	*I feel guilty and pressured about the mess.*

After brainstorming the list in the office, have your client rate each column—using the percentage of weight they assign to each side, from 0% to 100%—so that both sides add up to 100%. For example, if the benefits were rated at 40%, the costs would be rated at 60%.

This exercise will indicate which side should prevail, and it's no surprise that it's typically the benefits side. Since most individuals will assign a higher percentage to the benefits than to the costs, this technique often results in clients setting goals to end the procrastination.

☑ Behavioral Modification Techniques:
Use Behavioral Charts with Reinforcers

Most of us are aware of the charts that are used with children for the purpose of improving their behavior. The use of stickers, check marks, stars, and other tokens to reward improvement—following the principles of operant conditioning—can be quite effective with clients of all ages.

B. F. Skinner's operant conditioning theory has proven to be very effective in shaping new behaviors in both children and adults. When I was an instructor of psychology, I instructed my students to choose one behavioral goal (many of which turned out to be weight- or exercise-related) and record it in their semester diary. They found it quite motivational to devise a system of reinforcers to use when they completed a certain goal.

Use a calendar to list the specific goals of your clients and then implement a check system to indicate when an activity has been completed. Trading those checks in for a reward can help structure and motive your clients. The checks serve as a type of *token economy*, a notion developed by Skinner, in which the checks represent tokens that can be compiled and used for a tangible reward.

The resources section at the end of this chapter contains references to online behavioral charts and worksheets.

☑ DBT Technique: Behavioral Tracking Sheets and Diaries

The one area where we don't want our clients to procrastinate is in learning how to replace suicidal and self-harming behaviors with healthier ones. Obviously, there is a sense of urgency in this type of situation, and when helping a client replace this type of behavior, behavioral tracking sheets and diaries, essential to the Dialectical Behavior Therapy (DBT) approach, provide the answer. Linehan (1993), Van Dijk, (2012) and Mckay and Wood (2011) all have extensive examples of behavioral diaries and behavioral tracking sheets. All too often our clients procrastinate when attempting to replace self-destructive habits with healthier ones. This is especially the case when dealing with the borderline personality population. To respond to this concern, Linehan (1993) made behavioral tracking sheets an integral part of the DBT model. She views them as one of the essential between-session activities used to help clients gain new behaviors to regulate their actions and reduce their self-harming behavior.

The behavioral tracking sheets provide clients with a tool for logging their feelings and behaviors and noting their reactions and temptations related to urges to self-harm or use self-destructive behaviors. These sheets, which clients complete daily, help them to regulate their behavior and provide the therapist with important information about the client's behaviors and ability to self-regulate.

The common elements of daily monitoring are:

Identifying emotions
Strength of the emotions
Self-harm urges
Strength of the urges
Behaviors in reaction to strong emotions

In the handout section of this chapter are procrastination logs (Handouts 5.5, 5.6, and 5.7) to help your clients stay on track of their goals by Behavioral Tracking. The logs and diaries that are such a cornerstone of DBT treatment pinpoint unhealthy thoughts and cognitive distortions that interfere with proactivity.

☑ Behavioral Therapy Technique: Response Prevention

Response prevention is a useful strategy in working with clients to help them break the procrastination cycle. Response prevention is a technique used in behavioral therapy to reduce unwanted bad habits—or even compulsive behaviors—by removing the availability of the habitual responses during times of stress. Using this technique, your clients will be encouraged to pick areas in their lives in which they need to manage their environment differently by limiting their responses.

For example, if your clients want to stop smoking, they should not have cigarettes within their reach. If drinking wine has become a problem, you can suggest to them that they not have it in the house. If your client complains of having a weakness for Oreo cookies, you can suggest that response prevention (i.e., not buying the Oreos) might provide them the structure they need to make the commitment to discontinue their compulsive eating. Buying the Oreos and having them within reach is like expecting alcoholics to refrain from opening and drinking the bottle placed right in front of their eyes!

You can advise your clients that they may be able to rein in their procrastination by limiting the availability of diversions that take them away from behavior goals and new habits. For example, if they want to clean out the closets and are having a hard time getting motivated because they love going on Facebook, strategize with them how to limit their computer time. They might, for instance, shut the computer off for the rest of the evening, or limit the amount of time they allow themselves on the computer—or reward themselves with Facebook time after they finish cleaning the closet.

☑ Mini-Lesson: Helping Clients Become Proactive, Not Reactive

If you're proactive, you don't have to wait for circumstances or other people to create perspective expanding experiences. You can consciously create your own.

—Stephen Covey

Educating clients about leaders in the field of proactivity, such as Stephen Covey—can arm them with knowledge, which can be very motivational. Proactivity is the first of the seven traits that Stephen Covey used in formulating the best seller, *The Seven Habits of Highly Effective People*. Covey regarded those who took responsibility for their lives and did not blame others for their choices and action as highly effective. People who set their own goals and agendas are more likely to be successful. Covey uses the term "response-ability" as a play on the word *responsibility* to illustrate the importance of *choosing* how you respond in a situation, rather than *reacting* to others in a way that blames them for "making" you act or feel a certain way.

Highly proactive people recognize that they are responsible for their life and their behavior; they don't blame anyone else for derailing it or sidetracking them. They see their choices and behaviors as a product of their own conscious decisions, based on values, rather than the product of conditions outside of themselves.

Along these lines, I like to point out to my clients the distinction between the terms *proactive* and *reactive*. Proactive people focus on their own coping skills and not on how another person should behave. They focus on actualizing their own goals rather than judging what other people should or should not be doing, thus refusing to give up power to others.

☑ *Mini-Lesson: Choosing Victor Self-Talk*

Teaching your clients to differentiate between victim and victor self-talk will help them learn new skills and insights into their thinking, which can translate into increased self-empowerment. The following are examples of reactive *victim* language in contrast to proactive *victor* language. Providing your clients with this list can teach them skills to rephrase their *victim* thoughts into *victor* thoughts. Of course, reactive *victim talk* leads to procrastination, whereas proactive *victor talk* leads to taking control of your life. Procrastination self-talk is the type of talk that can truly make you your own worst enemy and prevent you from living the life you deserve to lead. It also makes you more reactive and powerless in the face of life events, rather than giving you the power to create what happens in your life.

Examples and Characteristics of . . .

Reactive *Victim* Self-Talk	Proactive *Victor* Self-Talk
Blaming others for your choices	Taking responsibility for your choices
"I should"	"I will"
"I have to"	"I choose to"
"I can't"	"I will and I can"
Prone to "stew"	Prone to "do"
Pessimistic	Optimistic
Feels controlled	Feels in control
"If only . . ."	"Only if . . ."
"He made me mad."	"I was mad when he said that."

The above comparison is an example of cognitive restructuring from victim self-talk to victor self-talk. The following techniques build on this mini-lesson to use various CBT cognitive restructuring techniques that are effective in overcoming procrastination.

☑ CBT Technique: The TIC-TOC Method

A catchy title for a CBT activity that helps clients identify the types of cognitive distortion they are prone to is the "TIC-TOC method." This is just one more tool in the therapeutic toolbox to help clients identify the unhealthy patterns of thinking that prevent them from making healthy life changes. David Burns (1999) uses the TIC-TOC method to illustrate how "TICs" (task-interfering cognitions) tend to interfere with thinking in healthier, proactive ways called "TOCS" (task-oriented cognitions). Utilizing the triple-column technique, he helps procrastinators identify the negative TICS and the types of cognitive distortion that result. The TOCs represent healthier and more action-oriented alternatives.

Below is a short example of common client TICS and TOCS. "Turning TICS Into TOCS" (Handout 5.2) will provide your clients a worksheet for identifying their TICS and TOCS between sessions.

TICS (Task-Interfering cognitions)	TOCS (Task-Oriented Cognitions)
I will never be able to feel better.	*That is an example of fortune telling. I will feel better once I become more active in my healing.*
I can't do anything right.	*That is an example of all-or-nothing thinking and overgeneralization. I do many things right; I am just frustrated that my progress seems slow.*
I'm just lazy.	*That is an example of labeling and self-blame. I have a hard time prioritizing.*

☑ CBT Technique: Playing the Devil's Advocate

Another cognitive strategy that Burns uses to overcome procrastination is the devil's advocate technique. Using this technique, the client writes down negative thoughts that undermine constructive action, such as "It's pointless to clean because the kids mess it up so quickly."

Once the list is complete, the therapist reads it while the client plays the devil's advocate in reversing these negative, irrational thoughts. Here is an example:

THERAPIST: *It's pointless to clean.*
CLIENT: *You will be able to relax and enjoy the house more when it is clean.*

This is also a great activity to be used in group sessions. Have your clients pair up; one reads the negative messages and the other plays the devil's advocate in refuting the negative thoughts.

☑ Activity: Help Your Clients Create an Action Plan Using SMART Goals

When my clients want to develop a game plan to overcome bad habits and overcome procrastination, I like to use the concept of SMART goals. I borrow this concept from the area of productivity, personal development, and management. This popular acronym is used quite often to depict the five characteristics of effective goal setting. Originally coined by management expert Peter Drucker and initially described in 1981 by George Doran in a business management journal, *Management Review*, SMART goals have become a cornerstone of the recipe for success. To employ SMART goals, your clients will first need some psychoeducation about what they are.

SMART goals are:

Specific. Be specific about what you want to achieve; a vague goal will be doomed to fail unless it is supported by specific goals to get there.

Measurable. Designate some criterion for measuring the success of your goals objectively so that you know when the goal has been reached.

Achievable. Goals must be attainable and realistic.

Relevant. Choose goals that you really care about, not something that seems pointless to you. Lack of relevance typically leads to procrastination.

Time-bound. Assigning target dates and time frames will make goals more limited in scope and easier to commit to than a goal with a vague timetable. Whether it is today, next week, a month from now, or a year from now, having goals that have a due date are easier to work toward.

Creating SMART goals with your clients by writing them out in session and making sure that both of you refer to them regularly is a solution-oriented approach to helping them make major changes in their lives without the procrastination factor. Make sure the goal is within their control. For example, having the goal of getting a job in three weeks is not completely within one's control. What is attainable is sending out 20 résumés and following up each with a phone call within three weeks. Thus, the key to using SMART goals is to focus on helping your clients choose a goal that they are completely empowered to fulfill and that does not depend on luck or happenstance.

In the case of a client who wants to lose weight, you would avoid the vague goal of just losing weight and make a game plan that serves as a blueprint for success. For example, bringing veggies to work for snacks is a positive action, while deciding not to buy snacks from the vending machines is a preventative goal.

Here is an example of how to create a plan for change with your clients using SMART goals.

Specific. To lose 20 pounds, I will attend Weight Watchers and take walks or go on the treadmill for a minimum of 20 minutes, four times per week.

Measurable. Weight Watchers will help me with this by having me go on the scale each time I attend meetings. I will also create an exercise diary/log to record how many times per week I walk and for how long.

Achievable. I will expect to lose weight gradually, ideally a pound or two a week. I will focus on sticking my plan and know that with increased exercise and less eating I will be moving in the right direction.

Relevant. I am committed to losing weight not because my parent or spouse is nagging me, but because I feel that weight loss will benefit me, both mentally and physically.

Time-bound. My goal is to lose a minimum of 2 pounds each month for the next 10 months, which is achievable based on my plan of action.

Now that your clients have established a goal, the next step is to help them create a plan that focuses on the day-to-day details of achieving their goal. Ensure that they break down the activity into small, manageable pieces. One reason why we procrastinate is that we do not break our goals into manageable segments.

For example, Dan, a 55-year-old insurance agent, was overwhelmed and immobilized by all the papers in his office, and he felt very inefficient and disorganized. The stress he was feeling was overwhelming, and having 30 years of files scattered around proved to be so daunting that he was getting very depressed and anxious just at the thought of going to work. He established a goal of cleaning his office in small steps, putting aside at least 20 minutes each day of the five-day workweek. He found that having this game plan in place resulted in more progress.

We also prioritized his to-do list in order of importance, making a hierarchy. After he was able to prioritize the list, he could check off each item as he accomplished it. The act of writing things down and monitoring progress serves as a reinforcer to many people. It also helps to include mini-reinforcements throughout the plan. Dan used reinforcers such as taking his wife to dinner once he completed cleaning out his two desks, which took a couple of weeks. Having a short-term celebration helped to motivate him, and he also found that by sharing his goal with another person, he was more likely to accomplish it.

This example helps to illustrate the elements of a successful PLAN:

Prioritize. Dan prioritized what needed to be done, then broke his tasks into smaller pieces that he was able to tackle for 20 minutes a day.

List. Dan created a list of the specific things he needed to do (the more specific, the better) and rated them in a hierarchy of what needed to be done first, second, and so forth. Handout 5.3 ("Hierarchy of Activities for Overcoming Procrastination") can be given to your clients so they can develop a hierarchy of activities to reach their goal, starting with the most desired goal on the top and going to the least desired goal on the bottom.

Action. Don't wait to get in the mood; as the Nike slogan states, "Just do it!" Dan committed himself to act on his list and monitored his progress by checking off each item as he completed it. Rather than allow himself to put tasks off, he took his plan seriously just like it was a job, "showing up" and "just doing it" consistent with his pre-determined schedule.

Note Progress. Have your clients note their progress in some form, whether by using checkmarks or some other reward, such as watching a TV show that they enjoy, after completing a task. Dan noted his progress by making checkmarks after tasks were completed. He also planned that 10 checkmarks would earn him a celebratory dinner out with his wife at a special restaurant. He also noted his progress verbally with his wife, enlisting her as an "accountability partner" to support his progress and boost his motivation.

In contemplating helping your clients to create SMART goals and have a PLAN, make sure you evaluate their readiness to change. SMART goals are not magical—they work only if your clients are ready to have them work. Prochaska and DiClemente's *Stages of Change*, which is the foundation of motivational interviewing, emphasizes the importance of being sensitive to whether or not the client is ready to change. According to their model, sometimes a client is in what is referred to as the "precontemplation" stage of change and therefore is not yet ready to commit to making changes. Therefore, what may appear to be procrastination is due to the fact that the client is not yet buying into the need to change.

Procrastination will certainly be an issue if the goals of the therapist differ from those of the client. A common example is that of alcohol abuse. All too often, clients who abuse alcohol may be in the precontemplation stage of change, during which they are not ready for change. If the therapist creates an agenda that the client does not share or find relevant, the client will often drop out of therapy. Any attempt to try to convince the client of what his or her goal should be will be doomed to fail if the client is not really ready for change.

Mini-Lesson: Food/Mood-Related Procrastination

One of the main reasons we procrastinate is that some habits are hard to break, especially when they relate to food and exercise. Food and mood are intertwined very closely. Educating our clients about the common link between *"low mood, more food"* is quite helpful. In fact, "Low mood, more food" may be at the core of why it is difficult for people who struggle with sadness and depression to lose weight and keep it off. As the title of Geneen Roth's landmark book on emotional eating—*When Food is Love* (1991)—suggests, food is not purely for sustenance or even pleasure; it becomes a way to feed ourselves love. This is especially true if we grew up in an unhealthy environment and used food as a way to comfort ourselves. Educating our clients about this connection, and providing resources such as Roth's book, to gain insight and overcome this cycle, can be very enlightening.

Because habits of emotional eating represent deep-seated feelings about our sense of self-worth and need for love, it is not surprising that diet habits are a tough nut to crack. Exploration of that deep-seated relationship between food and self-esteem and the need for love provides an avenue for therapeutic discussion. To further master this vicious cycle, the solution-oriented therapist needs some tools to help clients explore the food/mood/love connection. The "Food/Mood/Thought Diary" (Handout 5.4) will come in handy for situations in which your clients are struggling with emotional eating. It can help them to identify the thought and feeling triggers behind their emotional eating and help them focus on alternative behaviors.

☑ CBT TEchniques: Using Rewards and Reinforcements

Judith Beck focuses on helping clients recognize the toxic thoughts that sabotage their weight loss efforts in her book *The Beck Diet Solution*

(2008). One of her points in the book is how self-sabotaging thoughts can undermine following a healthy food plan. Examples of sabotaging thoughts are "I had a hard day, so I will treat myself," "I hate myself for eating what I shouldn't," and "I blew it, so I might as well have another piece of pie."

For a general systematic approach to the issue of dieting with a psychological focus, *The Beck Diet Solution* is an excellent guide to help clients change their toxic self-talk in relation to food. In the Beck Diet Solution, Judith Beck uses various reward charts and reinforcements to help readers develop strategies for losing weight. She also focuses on cognitive errors that undermine weight loss, and suggests to her readers that they create what she terms *advantage response cards* (see example below) to help them remember their reinforcements and goals and stay motivated.

Advantage response cards work best when clients make the commitment to review them regularly, at least a couple times a day, as they develop new habits. If they are not read, they won't work, and they need to be read regularly if they are to help clients break old habits and start new ones. Beck even suggests that clients include a card that reminds them to read their advantage response cards! These advantage response cards are a type of her CBT coping cards, which are basically note cards (or "cards" in electronic form) that clients make and look at to keep themselves grounded and focused on their goals.

Example of an Advantage Response Card

I know I will feel better about the way I look if I stick to my diet and exercise plan.
I will be able to fit into my prepregnancy clothes again.
I will have more energy.
I will look better at my son's wedding.

In *The Beck Diet Solution*, Judith Beck also provides practical lists, such as a scheduling chart to help clients track their activities from morning until night. After reviewing the chart, clients create a new one to prioritize and change their activities to suit their new goals and lifestyle plan. Thus, having a priority chart that prioritizes activities helps shape new habits and behaviors. An example of this focus is found in "Hierarchy of Activities for Overcoming Procrastination" (Handout 5.3), in which clients rank their behavioral goals in order of importance and track their progress each day of the week. The success of *The Beck Diet Solution* is an example of the importance of bibliotherapy in helping your clients stay focused and motivated to change. By knowing important resources to offer them, you can help them maintain progress between sessions. Most therapists underestimate the importance of bibliotherapy and using diaries and handouts between sessions. These resources make treatment much more effective, and progress comes more quickly when clients use them at home and review them in session. The resources section at the end of this chapter will list other books, links, and other materials that may be useful in helping your clients overcome procrastination.

In the next section, we will focus on how to help your clients establish a clearer vision of their goals and values.

☑ ACT Visualization: Establishing a Life Vision and Life Values

Part of the difficulty in treating procrastination issues is that our clients may not have a clear vision of what their values and vision for themselves truly are. Acceptance and Commitment Therapy (ACT) emphasizes the importance of helping clients clarify and visualize their values and vision so that their actions can represent a commitment to those values. Values are important in ACT, as these values are seen as guides to action. The rationale is that once a client is clear about goals and values, procrastination will likely be much less of a factor. This is because committed action will be guided by a personal sense of values and vision.

ACT makes liberal use of metaphors to make points. One of the best-known metaphors used by ACT founder Steven Hayes is "monsters on the bus." In this analogy, the individual is the bus driver and various monsters are directing the driver where to go, causing the driver to veer from the scheduled route. These monsters sabotage the driver by saying negative thoughts, and the driver is so influenced by all the monsters that he veers off course. Thus, the bus ends up going in the wrong direction and the driver is not in control of the bus—the monsters are.

The point of this analogy is that if clients are not guided by their values and vision, they will not be directed in their behavior and will not have a strong sense of direction to meet personal goals. If your clients do not have a sense of values-driven commitment, the monsters in their head will interfere with their getting anywhere. Hayes makes the point that the more you are committed to and certain of your direction, the less you will listen to the negative monsters that sidetrack you from your sense of goal and purpose.

☑ CBT Technique: Goal Setting With Pie Charts

Once your clients have focused on their values, life goals, and vision for themselves, it is time for them to set some specific goals. Goal setting is an important aspect of overcoming procrastination; it is easier to take action when you have a plan and a direction. One popular CBT method makes use of the old-fashioned pie chart. Pie charts help clients visualize how they spend their time and how they want to spend their time as they prioritize their goals.

Judith Beck calls this method the pie technique. She suggests that helping clients see their ideas in graphic form helps them to understand where they focus their attention and where they want to focus that attention. She suggests using the pie technique when your clients need help in specifying what their problem areas are and what their goals are to change them. She uses the example of a student who got a low grade on a test and charted the reasons for this, assigning various percentages to unpreparedness, depression, test difficulty, and so forth. Pie charts can provide a great visual. This technique can be used in groups, where participants can compare their charts with those of others.

This pie chart visualization is commonly used by productivity specialists, work–life balance experts, and business consultants—not just therapists—to help people clarify their present life choices compared to what they would like their lives to be. Two charts are often used, as seen below, with one pie chart indicating how the client spends his or her time currently and the other representing how the client would ideally apportion his or her time. Seeing the visualization helps clients to specify what changes they want to make in their lives. Often, this brings home the fact that too much time is spent on some parts of life at the exclusion of other parts.

There are many ways to separate the categories, and the model below is only an example.

Joe was a middle-aged manager with work–life balance issues. Here is his chart:

How I Slice My Life Chart

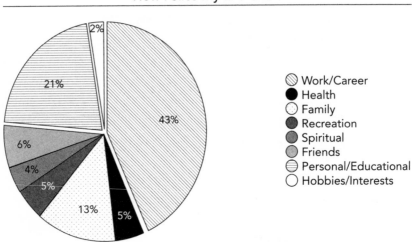

As you can see, Joe has pretty much neglected personal self-care activities in response to the demands of career and nighttime graduate school, leaving little time for family and almost no time for friends and church.

As I looked at Joe's goals with him, he then made another pie chart based on how he would ideally like to apportion his life. It looked like this:

How I Would Like to Slice My Life Chart

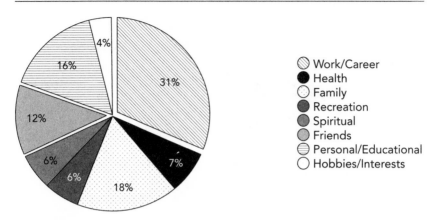

Work/Career
Health
Family
Recreation
Spiritual
Friends
Personal/Educational
Hobbies/Interests

Joe decided to allow himself more time to get involved with self-care and spend more time with his family. He decided to take fewer night classes and made an effort not to bring work home.

☑ Life Wheel Activity: Finding a Life Balance

Another great use of the pie chart is as a life wheel. The life wheel has as its slices various areas of life, and each one is rated from 1 to 10 based on how much these areas are focused on. The number 1 is at the center and 10 is in the rim, and clients are asked to place a dot somewhere between 1 and 10 indicating how much energy they put into these various areas of their life. Then, when the dots are connected, it becomes evident where your clients are focusing their attention and where adjustments may need to be made for them to achieve more of a life balance.

☑ CBT Activity: The Procrastination Pie Chart

Another use of a pie chart is as a tool for focusing on thoughts instead of actual behaviors. It can help your clients identify reasons for their procrastination. Take the example of a client who was dissatisfied with her present job but was immobilized about making efforts to start looking for a new one. Although she had very solid work experience and seemed to be quite marketable in office work, she felt paralyzed to even try.

A Life Wheel

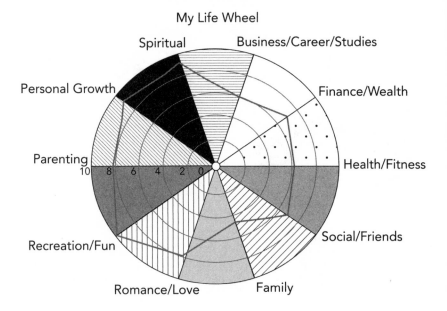

My Life Wheel

We first listed reasons why she procrastinated:

Fear of rejection
Fear of present company finding out she is looking
Feelings of insecurity about being "good enough"
Fear of failure and then needing to sell her home
Lack of time
"I don't like change"
Too depressed
Will miss some coworkers

I then had my client put a percentage by how strong her thought was for each item, rating each thought from 1 to 100.

Fear of rejection: 20%
Fear of present company finding out she is looking: 10%
Feeling of insecurity about being "good enough": 30%

Fear of failure and then needing to sell her home: 35%
Lack of time: 25%
"I don't like change": 20%
Too depressed: 40%
Will miss some coworkers: 10%

Her pie chart looked like this.

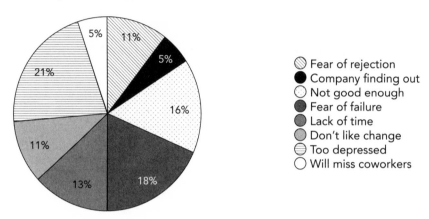

Fear of rejection
Company finding out
Not good enough
Fear of failure
Lack of time
Don't like change
Too depressed
Will miss coworkers

The visualization above was striking to my client and helped her see how unhealthy thoughts were holding her back from living a happier and more productive life. It helped convince her to start putting more effort into overcoming her distorted fear of failure, fear of rejection, and low self-esteem. Once she spent more time reading self-help materials on overcoming low self-esteem and began filling out her logs and work-sheets regularly, she was finally able to get motivated to start looking for another job.

A Toolkit of Metaphors for Overcoming Procrastination

The following metaphorical objects can help your clients overcome pro-crastination.

> **A can.** Clients can leave a can at their desk at work or at home to help them remember to have a "can do" attitude.

A circle. Have a circle cut out of poster board to remind your clients about the life wheel and the pie chart exercises to help them clarify their values and goals.

Nike logo. A Nike swish logo can remind your clients to "just do it!"

Post-it note. This reminds your client to make notes, write things down, and track their behavior.

Gold star sticker. This serves as a reminder of the importance of reinforcements in shaping behavior.

Can you and your client think of more metaphors? This is a great group activity!

Therapeutic Takeaways

☑ Although some element of procrastination is common for most people, procrastination can significantly impede healthy life adjustment when clients are already impaired by symptoms of depression and anxiety.

☑ Clients can learn skills and techniques to limit their procrastination. There are various methods from both Behavior Therapy and Cognitive Behavior Therapy that are effective in helping clients overcome procrastination. It is important for therapists to be aware of various strategies that offer structure and education to their clients as they attempt to overcome procrastination.

☑ Some of the methods we can teach our clients use behavioral conditioning principles of reinforcement to encourage productive behavior. Filling out behavioral tracking sheets, keeping logs, completing worksheets, developing a hierarchy of goals, and making alternative response cards are some examples of how clients can stay motivated between sessions.

☑ Strategies for goal setting, like pie charts, aid clients in being more proactive and clarify areas they will need to address to become more successful in meeting their goals.

☑ Goals are most likely to be accomplished when they are SMART goals.

Handouts

The following worksheets will help your clients develop anti-procrastination skills. These handouts have been referred to in the body of this chapter. As a general guideline, handouts and assignments are given to your clients at the end of the session. Make sure you leave ample time to go over your expectations for use of the selected handout.

When assignments are given out, it is important to follow up with your clients at the beginning of the next session by reviewing and discussing their homework with them. Going over the homework is an essential aspect of being a solution-oriented therapist.

Note: All handouts in the book are available for download on my website by following the link below: http://www.belmontwellness.com/ultimate-solution-handouts/

Handout 5.1: Common Myths About Procrastination

Myth 1: People who procrastinate are just plain lazy.

Calling someone "lazy" is an example of the cognitive error of labeling. However, when people feel stuck and are inactive, they often think of themselves as lazy, which makes them even more self-deprecatory and causes them to be more stuck. In reality, procrastination is a sign of deep-seated issues such as fear of failure, perfectionism, depression, and lack of clarification of goals and values.

Myth 2: For constructive action, it's best to wait to "get in the mood."

We go to work or school even if we don't feel like it. Waiting for being in the mood is like waiting for the weather to change—sometimes it takes a long time. We can act constructively even if we feel depressed and anxious, and if we wait to feel better, we are dependent on things largely outside our control. Actually, once people take action, they often feel better—so action often comes before an elevated mood.

Myth 3: It's best to just "get the job done" rather than do it over a period of time.

Studies have shown that taking a big task and breaking it into small pieces will actually increase the chances of getting it done. People who wait to have the chunk of time they need to do a job and "bite the bullet" might never actually get the chunk of time they want. Chipping away in smaller blocks of time will generally get the job done. (How do you eat an elephant? One bite at a time!)

Myth 4: Rewarding yourself for taking action is a form of bribery.

Actually, reinforcement helps us change. Bribes have a negative connotation, and there is nothing negative about using the principles of reinforcement. Many studies have documented the motivation that reinforcement provides as we work toward our goals.

Handout 5.2: Turning TICS Into TOCS

The following is a 2-page worksheet for identifying your task-interfering thoughts, the types of distortion behind those thoughts, and rational alternatives. This is based on the work of author David Burns.

TICS (Task-Interfering Cognitions)	Types of Cognitive Distortion	TOCS (Task-Oriented Cognitions)
Example: "I'll never feel better."	Fortune telling, all-or-nothing thinking, sense of futility	"I will feel better once I become more active in my healing."

Sample Types of Faulty-Thinking Habits

1. **Catastrophizing.** You label things are horrible and awful instead of unfortunate and disappointing. *Example: "This is HORRIBLE!"*
2. **Fortune telling.** You think you can predict the future. *Example: "I'll never find anyone who will be interested in me. I'll be alone the rest of my life."*
3. **Black-and-white thinking.** You make all-or-nothing assumptions. *Example: "Men are liars."*
4. **Personalization.** You blame yourself for things out of your control. *Example: "I am to blame for my child's issues."*
5. **Jumping to conclusions.** You make assumptions and regard them as fact. *Example: "He told me he couldn't come to the party because he just doesn't like me."*
6. **Labeling.** You label yourself and other instead of being specific. *Example: Instead of saying " I made a mistake," you label yourself a "failure" or a "loser."*
7. **Magnification.** You make mountains out of molehills. *Example: "This is the worst day of my life"*
8. **Minimization.** You deny things are an issue when they are. *Example: You say "It's not a big deal" (when it really is) or "I don't care" (when you really do).*
9. **Mental filter.** You focus on one negative detail and not the whole picture, discounting the positives. *Example: "I am ugly because of my large nose."*
10. **"Should" statements.** You make self-downing judgments that keep you feeling down and stuck. *Example: "I should be able to get more done."*
11. **Sense of futility.** You assume things are futile and pointless. You feel doomed to fail. *Example: "Why even try?"*

Handout 5.3: Hierarchy of Activities for Overcoming Procrastination

Rank goals for the week in order of difficulty, 1 being the most difficult and 10 being the least difficult. Leave a check mark by the days you worked on each goal. This worksheet will help you prioritize your to-do list so you can stay on track.

Hierarchy of Goals and Activities

	Most Challenging Goal	S	M	T	W	T	F	S	Progress Notes
1									
2									
3									
4									
5									
6									
7									
8									
9									
10									
	Least Challenging Goal								

Handout 5.4: Food/Mood/Thought Diary

Use a food/mood/thought log daily or weekly to keep track of any sabotaging food choices. This will help you to identify the moods and unhealthy thoughts behind your unhealthy food choices. By developing awareness, you will become more successful in replacing old habits with new ones.

Date	Time	Unhealthy Food Choice	Mood	Thoughts	Alternative Responses: Thought and Behavior

NOTES FOR DEVELOPING NEW SKILL HABITS

_____

_____

_____

_____

Handout 5.5: Procrastination Log #1

Using Handout 5.6 as a model, use this form to help you overcome procrastination and take action!

Something I Am Procrastinating On	
Negative Emotions	Positive Emotions
Strength of Negative Emotions 1 2 3 4 5 6 7 8 9 10 Low　　　　　　　　High	Strength of Positive Emotions 1 2 3 4 5 6 7 8 9 10 Low　　　　　　　　High
Identify Negative Beliefs	Challenge With Positive Beliefs
Type of Thinking Error	Healthier Thought
Certainty of Your Beliefs 1 2 3 4 5 6 7 8 9 10 Low　　　　　　　　High	Certainty of Your Beliefs 1 2 3 4 5 6 7 8 9 10 Low　　　　　　　　High
Unhealthy Reactions	Healthy Reactions
Cost/Benefit Analysis: Unhealthy Coping	Cost/Benefit Analysis: Healthy Coping
My Conclusions and Goals	

Handout 5.6: Procrastination Log #1, Completed

Something I Am Procrastinating On
Would like to exercise five times per week for 40 minutes

Negative Emotions	Positive Emotions
Discouraged, unmotivated	Hopeful

Strength of Negative Emotions	Strength of Positive Emotions
_____X_____ 1 2 3 4 5 6 7 8 9 10 Low High	_____X_____ 1 2 3 4 5 6 7 8 9 10 Low High

Identify Negative Beliefs	Challenge With Positive Beliefs
Why bother? I am so out of shape and heavy. I'll never be thin and fit.	I will start feeling better if I go in the right direction.

Type of Thinking Error	Healthier Thought
All-or-nothing thinking, fortune telling	There is hope if I chip away gradually and exercise even 10 minutes a day to start.

Certainty of Your Beliefs	Certainty of Your Beliefs
X_____ 1 2 3 4 5 6 7 8 9 10 Low High	_____X_____ 1 2 3 4 5 6 7 8 9 10 Low High

Unhealthy Reactions	Healthy Reactions
Putting it off Avoiding work; watching TV	Taking some small steps; taking a short walk

Cost/Benefit Analysis: Unhealthy Coping	Cost/Benefit Analysis: Healthy Coping
Too much work! I have no time.	Benefits: Feeling better; feeling proud of myself, manage time

My Conclusions and Goals
I need to make my plan easier. I will start with 10 minutes a day and work up to 40.

Handout 5.6: Procrastination Log #2

*Date:*_____

1. Procrastination example

_____

_____

2. Emotional responses

_____

_____

3. Degree of negative stress   LOW 1 2 3 4 5 6 7 8 9 10 HIGH

4. Unhealthy thoughts

_____

_____

    Certainty of beliefs   LOW 1 2 3 4 5 6 7 8 9 10 HIGH

5. Type of thinking distortion

_____

_____

6. Healthy thoughts

_____

_____

    Certainty of beliefs   LOW 1 2 3 4 5 6 7 8 9 10 HIGH

7. Unhealthy reactions

_____

_____

8. Healthy reactions

_____

_____

9. My overall values that I am committed to

_____

_____

10. Specific Smart Goals I am setting

_____

_____

11. Example of the TIC TOC approach

_____

_____

12. Costs/benefits of my healthy and unhealthy thinking

_____

_____

13. Goal for overcoming procrastination

_____

_____

Recommended Resources

Self-Help Books

The Beck Diet Solution: Train Your Brain to Think Like a Thin Person
Judith S. Beck
The Feeling Good Handbook
David D. Burns
When Food Is Love: Exploring the Relationship Between Eating and Intimacy
Geneen Roth

Books With DBT Diaries and Tracking Sheets

Skills Training Manual for Treating Borderline Personality Disorder
Marsha M. Linehan
The Dialectical Behavior Therapy Diary: Monitoring Your Emotional Regulation Day by Day
Matthew McKay & Jeffrey C. Wood
DBT Made Simple: A Step-by-Step Guide to Dialectical Behavior Therapy
Sheri Van Dijk

Self-Help Procrastination Inventories

(Anti-procrastination client worksheet)
http://sourcesofinsight.com/how-to-use-an-antiprocrastination-sheet/
The Procrastination Test
David D. Burns, *The Feeling Good Handbook*, 1999, p. 171

Self-Help Worksheets and Links

(DBT diary cards)
http://www.dbtselfhelp.com/html/diary_cards1.html
http://www.mydailydbt.com/2012/12/printable-dbt-diary-card.html
Mind Tools
"Overcoming Procrastination"
http://www.mindtools.com/pages/article/newHTE_96.htm

"The Wheel of Life: Finding Balance in Your Life"
    http://www.mindtools.com/pages/article/newHTE_93.htm

Psychology Tools

(Worksheets, diaries, behavior charts, and tracking sheets)
    http://www.psychologytools.org/download-therapy-worksheets
    .html

Therapist Aid

(Worksheets and behavior charts)
    http://www.therapistaid.com/therapy-worksheets/none/none

CHAPTER SIX

The Conflict Solution
Improving Problematic Relationships

One of the major issues that prompt clients to seek therapy is conflict in relationships. Marital problems, interpersonal issues at work, difficulties with raising children, family disagreements, difficulties in dating relationships, and disputes with friends and neighbors are just a sampling of the myriad situations in which conflict arises. Few of us were ever taught about relationship skills in school; therefore, healthy communication practices will be one of the most important skills you can ever teach your clients.

Even if our clients' presenting problems are not initially regarded as problems in their relationships, effective therapy invariably uncovers the toll that our clients' individual presenting problems takes on those close to them. For example, clients who are depressed, angry, or anxious will understandably be unable to keep those symptoms isolated from their relationships with others. Conflicts with coworkers, friends, family members, and significant others are all fallouts from individual problems being played out in the social arena. For example, clients whose anger stems from early childhood issues are more likely to be insensitive and egocentric in dealing with others in their lives at present. These angry clients often tend to be more aggressive in their communication and are often poor listeners, lacking empathy for and sensitivity to those around them. In such cases, aggressive communication is actually an expression of deep-seated pain, disguised as obnoxiousness and arrogance. Likewise, clients who are depressed might withdraw from social support and connectedness, causing conflict with others due to their apathy and distancing from others. For these clients, non-assertive, indirect communication is more likely to occur, putting a strain on their relationships with others and limiting their ability for intimacy.

Conversely, just as it is common for individual clients to end up working on their relationship problems when they come in to work on personal problems, it is not uncommon for clients to enter marital or family therapy to find that along with improving their relationship issues, they need to work on "fixing" themselves. Often, relationship problems are symptoms of individual issues being played out in a relationship forum.

In sum, no clients' presenting problem can be seen in isolation of their relationships with others. Thus, regardless of the reasons why clients seek counseling, it is important to focus the on communication and conflict resolution skills for almost every client. After all, we are social creatures and do not live in isolation.

Sometimes the conflict in communication is not due to overt conflict with others but rather with the demons inside your clients' own heads. Fear of saying the wrong thing or saying something stupid, risking disapproval and ridicule, triggers all types of communication issues such as shyness and social phobia. Many times we need to provide clients with tools to develop the confidence to speak up without fear of being rejected or judged. Psychoeducation on how to communicate more effectively and confidently is based on teaching them the three basic types of communication: *assertive, nonassertive,* and *aggressive.* "The Three Types of Communication" handout (Handout 6.2) has long remained among my most frequently used ones, and has helped me introduce to my clients the basics of healthy communication. Most have found that differentiating between the three types of communication eye opening.

To provide a more detailed analysis of the differences between the three communication types, I use handouts like "Comparing the Three Types of Communication" (Handout 6.3). This is one of my "go-to" handouts whenever my clients have interpersonal communication issues—which is very often! An understanding of the important differences between healthy assertive behavior and the unhealthy reactions of both

175

aggressive and nonassertive behavior is crucial in dealing with difficult relationships as well as one's own conflict-ridden self-talk.

There are well-documented mental health benefits that go along with maintaining strong interpersonal connections. Many studies have shown that a strong supportive network is one of the fundamentals of life satisfaction, and in fact, widening your social network as you age—rather than allowing it to shrink—is correlated with happiness and health later in life.

In the example below, I illustrate some important interventions in the area of communication and conflict. By having a varied supply of communication worksheets, handouts, and activities in my toolbox, I have been able to offer clients skills to last a lifetime. Even though navigating through relationships can be complicated, being more assertive and dealing effectively with the aggressive behavior of others becomes much easier when clients learn tips to recognize the difference between assertive and aggressive behavior.

Forty-two-year old Ben was depressed and simmering with anger at the way his wife treated him. In retaliation, he tuned her out and refused to carry out some of his responsibilities at home, and then felt more ashamed and depressed. He felt he could never win with his wife, and internalized his anger. He himself had grown up in a volatile household and learned to survive by keeping his feelings to himself. He was afraid of anger, especially his own, and tried to suppress any such feelings for fear that he would erupt. To prevent himself from erupting, he carried himself in a very quiet, soft-spoken, and rather expressionless manner. What had been a survival skill under his volatile parent's radar when he was younger was now leading to marital discord. Ben's much more emotional wife had become highly frustrated at his lack of emotional connectedness and his tendency to retreat, which triggered her to blow up more.

Learning that anger does not have to be aggressive and that it can be expressed positively was a welcome relief for Ben. The anger he had known from his parents and wife had not been expressed positively. By realizing that anger was not an emotion to be suppressed and feared, he was ready to learn new skills to manage his anger and speak up more.

The Conflict Solution

The first step in Ben's treatment was to provide him with psychoeducation. In the treatment tips section, I will start with the first psychoeducational lesson that I teach clients as a basis for understanding the three types of communication: *assertive*, *nonassertive*, and *aggressive*.

Treatment Tips

☑ Mini-Lesson: Healthy Communication Basics

We communicate all the time, yet the guidelines for healthy communication are not universally learned in the same way. Most of our clients experience some type of relationship conflicts, and since so much of our work and life success is contingent on effective communication, teaching them the guidelines of healthy communication can help them improve their lives considerably. Unhealthy relationships are the unfortunate fallout from a lack of knowledge leading to miscommunication.

It is not uncommon for people to think they are acting in a healthy assertive fashion when they are really acting quite aggressively. All too often our clients might start out assertively, but, if they do not get their way, escalate to aggressive behavior, and feel justified in escalating to aggression because they did not get the results they wanted. The rule of thumb is that if your goal is aggressive, such as to get others to change their mind, then aggressive behavior results even if the communication starts out calmly. All too often our clients feel justified in escalating to being aggressive because they feel misunderstood and want to change the other person. They truly believe it is for the other person's own good and feel justified in their aggressive communication because they feel that they are *right* and the other person is *wrong*. The rule of thumb is that if a person's goal is to change others it is aggressive communication. When the goal becomes less about *expressing* oneself and more about *impressing* a point, trouble arises. I often remind my clients that they can change someone's reality, but they can *never* change their perceptions! With aggressive behavior the goal is all too often to change perceptions, which can prove futile!

To teach your clients how to keep from falling into common communication traps, below are some basic ways to identify the three types of communication. This knowledge will help your clients express their thoughts and feelings constructively. In the handouts section, I have included some of my favorite communication handouts to bolster this mini-lesson.

To start off, teach your clients the difference between the three types of communication: *aggressive*, *nonassertive*, and *assertive*.

THE AGGRESSIVE MOTTO: *I'M OK—YOU'RE NOT!*

Aggressive behavior focuses on "you" statements, in which an individual tells others how they "should" be. It is disrespectful and controlling, with the goal being to change the other person instead of merely asking for a change. Thoughts are honest and direct, but also blunt and tactless, lacking sensitivity to the other person. Aggressive communication is designed to dominate, control, prove how right one is, or "get back at someone," even if it's silent aggression—that is, the cold shoulder or "silent treatment."

Payoffs: A sense of superiority, power, and control; a sense of righteousness; fulfillment of the need to be right, seem strong, get your way, and blame others

Emotional cost: Aggressive individuals feel angry, indignant, alienated, lonely, and they hold grudges.

Goal: To change others, to get your way, to prove the other person wrong and yourself right, to be an authority and superior.

THE NONASSERTIVE MOTTO: *YOU'RE OK—I'M NOT!*

Nonassertive behavior allows others to infringe on one's rights due to the individual's fear of making waves and receiving disapproval. It is a "people-pleasing" mode of communication in which you let others intimidate you and you feel inferior and insecure, wanting approval from others at the expense of your own. Worry about what people think and not wanting to make waves takes its toll, leading to anxiety and depression.

Payoffs: Avoidance of conflict, feelings of greater approval from others, feelings of greater safety.

Emotional cost: Nonassertive individuals feel needy, insecure, anxious, powerless, and fearful.

Goal: To be liked, to get the approval of others, to stay "below the radar."

THE ASSERTIVE MOTTO: *I'M OK—YOU'RE OK!*

Assertive behavior is the happy medium and the ideal type of communication, and is characterized by "I" statements in which everyone's rights and needs are respected. Communication is direct, calm, confident, honest—but tactful, unlike aggressive communication, in which tact and finesse are not valued. Assertive individuals express and assert their rights, needs, and desires without needing the approval of others. Their own self-approval is also valued. They respect others and respect themselves too.

Payoffs: Self-confidence, self-expression, honest and close relationships

Emotional benefits: Assertive individuals feel confident, secure, empowered, calm, and friendly.

Goal: To express, not impress! To improve, not prove! The underlying desire is to be open and foster closeness.

☑ Mini-Lesson: Communication Skills 101

I support my clients' communication skills with psychoeducational lessons and handouts over the course of counseling. With Ben, the client I talked about earlier in the chapter, I reviewed Handout 6.2 ("The Three Types of Communication"), Handout 6.3 ("Comparing the Three Types of Communication") and Handout 6.1 ("Common Myths About Conflict") with him to dispel some of his misunderstandings about communication and conflict. Worksheets such as "Turn *You* Statements Into *I* Statements" (Handout 6.4) helped us focus on turning Ben's own *You* statements into *I* statements. I emphasized to Ben that even thinking in *You* statements in one's self-talk often result in aggressive *you* statements with others because the thinking is aggressive.

Your clients will likely need a lot of practice transforming *You* statements into *I* statements. You will need to clarify with your client that even if you start a statement with *I*, it doesn't mean you're home free! There are many *You* statements that start with *I*. For example, consider this statement: "I think you stink!" Conversely, you can use the word *You* without it being a *you* statement, such as in "You mean a lot to me."

Because healthy communication is such an important topic, I have many communication tools in my therapeutic toolbox. Additional sheets, such as "My Communication Diary" (Handout 6.9), give clients other opportunities to track their progress and continue to work on their skills.

For enacting role-plays with clients, one of the most helpful sheets is the "Checklist for Assertive Communication" (Handout 6.8). In this sheet, I have outlined a checklist of assertive communication hallmarks, and I emphasize the importance of making sure the communication goal is an assertive one. All too often, well-meaning clients want to convince someone of their point of view, and inadvertently get aggressive since they are trying to change the other person—whether it is their minds or their actions. The first item in the checklist is to evaluate if the goal is an assertive one; an assertive goal would be geared toward expressing oneself and not impressing upon changing others. Another item on the checklist is to have clients determine their individual rights and weigh them against their corresponding responsibilities. "Bill of Rights: Basic Human Rights and Corresponding Responsibilities" (Handout 6.6) offers clients some assistance in identifying their rights, such as the right to say no, the right to ask for help, and the right to express one's feelings, including anger. These rights, of course, need to be weighed against one's responsibilities to others, such as being tactful and empathetic, being caring and considerate, and expressing anger without being aggressive. "My Communication-Tracking Log" (Handout 6.10) will help your client put all their learning together in one behavioral tracking form to be completed between sessions.

I used all these type of sheets as guides for role-playing and practicing new assertiveness skills with Ben. It didn't take too long for Ben to speak more openly with his wife, and to assert his needs rather than keep them in. He began to feel happier and less inhibited, and he felt less and less angry, and was less afraid of her anger.

Ben was surprised that even though he set more limits on his wife's aggressive behavior, they got along better because he no longer enabled her aggression. Despite the fact that she herself was not in treatment, by his reports, her behavior also improved, as Ben was no longer enabling it. It turns out that she didn't know aggressive behavior was wrong, and once she read the materials he would bring home and talked with him about it, she also learned to change her *You* statements into *I* statements in many situations. Ben learned that the feeling of anger was not undesirable, and learned not to confuse it with aggressive behavior.

These very practical psychoeducational lessons, backed up by the various communication skills handouts that Ben found so helpful, are invaluable in the case of couple counseling. When I see couples, I am struck by how they almost invariably come in to the session thinking that it is their spouse who is the difficult one. After they get some education on communication skills, they often realize that they both were being difficult—at least the ones whose marriages have a chance. I often joke with my clients that in "dealing with difficult people," make sure the difficult one is not you! Clients are often amazed to find that they are also the difficult one!

In working with argumentative couples, I usually allow them to argue for only a few minutes before stopping them. I ask them who they think is the really difficult one, and invariably they point to each other. Instead of convincing them that they both are being difficult—after all, it takes two to engage in an argument—I let them discover that for themselves, as people learn better from lessons they find out on their own.

To help them decide who indeed is the difficult one, I pull out my sheets on conflict and communication. Many times, the remainder of the session is a skill-building session. So that nobody feels picked on, I show them handouts such as "The Three Types of Communication" and "Comparing the Three Types of Communication" (Handouts 6.2 and 6.3), teaching them about the types of communication, and then I ask them how they would characterize their own behavior in that argument. If I told them they were acting aggressive, they could get resistant and feel judged. Yet, if I show them the handouts, they always get it right. By deciding that their communication was aggressive, they demonstrate that they can now identify the differences and know what they need to change, such as turning *You* statements into *I* statements. Identifying their own behavior with the help of the handouts does not put them on the defensive as it much easier for them to accept and understand the hallmarks of healthy versus unhealthy communication by seeing it clearly on the paper. After they look at the guidelines for aggressive communication and identify their own behavior, it is easier to refer to these points during role plays in session and helps them act more assertively in their personal relationships.

Jerry and Dana had been in counseling for a few months before coming to my office, but they decided to try out a new therapist since they got tired of going to her office to argue. They figured they already did a good job on their own arguing, and didn't need anybody watching. They were taken aback that after they had argued a couple of minutes, I stopped them, and instead of letting them go on, I pulled out some handouts to teach them about communication basics. I saw them almost every week for about six months, and I never saw them argue again. Besides giving them the handouts previously mentioned, I furthered their education with "Aggressive Behavior: Reasons, Payoffs and Consequences" (Handout 6.5), "Bill of Rights: Basic Human Rights and Corresponding Responsibilities" (Handout 6.6), and "Communication Basics" (Handout 6.7). With these handouts, they explored in more depth the reasons and payoffs for their conflict, and were able to realize that although it was fine for them to stand up for their own rights, they had corresponding responsibilities to treat others with respect.

It is interesting to note that prior to counseling, each of them thought that it was the other who was the difficult one! They learned that, most of all, even if the other was difficult, they did not need to follow suit and let the other set the tone for their behavior. Just as they told their children, "it doesn't matter who starts it—it matters who ends it!"

☑ Mini-Lesson: Active Listening

One of the main points that Jerry and Dana learned well is that hearing is not the same thing as listening, even though those terms are often used interchangeably. When we think of communication, we often think of what we say, not how we listen. But good listening skills are one of the hallmarks of good communication and just as important as what you say.

Although hearing and listening go hand in hand and complement one another, in times of interpersonal conflict, the difference between them cannot be more apparent. Educating your clients regarding the difference will be helpful to them as they deal with problems in their relationships.

The following are some major differences between hearing and listening. These are a great springboard to use for role play when working with clients to improve their listening skills; it is especially effective in a couple's session.

Hearing is passive and is the act of merely taking in audible sounds.
Listening is active and requires empathy, skill, and interpretation.

Hearing without listening can lead to arguments and defensiveness, with the goal of proving that you are right.
Listening is not defensive—it is about trying to understand the other, not to prove yourself.

Hearing shows that you care about yourself and what you want to say in response.
Listening shows that you care about the other person.

Hearing leads you to accept things at face value without interpretation.
Listening helps you read between the lines.

Hearing leads to assumptions and misperceptions.
Listening helps you summarize, clarify, and clear up misperceptions.

Hearing leads to verbal as well as nonverbal aggression and non-assertion.

Listening leads to healthy, assertive relationships.

☑ Activity: Role Play for Assertiveness

Now that your client has a fundamental understanding of communication and has learned the difference between listening and hearing, together you can put the learning into practice through role play. Role play is a staple of the Cognitive Behavior Therapy (CBT), Dialectical Behavior Therapy (DBT), and other popular approaches. There is no shortage of variations of role play that you can conduct with your clients; I use role play in almost every session that addresses problematic interpersonal relationships to help my clients practice the skills they learned in session. I play their spouse, child, coworker, parent, etc., and it is not uncommon for us to switch places if I want to model assertive responses. Role plays don't even have to represent real people in your clients' lives; they can be an enactment of a client's negative thoughts or worst fears, for instance. You and you client can take turns acting out both sides of the thought, one proposing the thought and the other disputing it. I make the point that it is just as important to talk assertively to yourself as it is to others, as aggressive self-talk leads to low self-esteem, depression, and anxiety.

In groups, role play with fellow group members to practice assertiveness skills is invaluable, especially for shy or anxious clients who have trouble expressing themselves in their daily lives. Often I have group members go into small groups of 3 or 4 and they take turns role playing situations from their lives, gaining valuable feedback from the group on how they came across.

Role play is most effective when clients use relevant handouts as a guide to evaluating whether their communication was effective. The handouts at the end of this section are a good springboard for learning about good communication and practicing it. Handouts are invaluable in helping clients understand their ineffective communications in a non-judgmental, matter-of-fact way, limiting the possibility of defensiveness.

It is also helpful for clients to see the concepts they are learning in black and white; this often makes a bigger impression on them.

"The Three Types of Communication" (Handout 6.2) and "Comparing the Three Types of Communication" (Handout 6.3) are good handouts to start with. I also use the "Checklist for Assertive Communication" (Handout 6.8) to evaluate role plays in session. For example, first on the list is "Ask yourself, 'What is my goal?' Make sure it is an assertive goal." This is important because all too often people do not realize that their goal is to change someone else, and therefore is aggressive. Asking for a change is fine—having the expectation that someone "should" change is another thing. Handout 6.8 helps structure role plays and can be used as a guide when clients practice communication outside of the session.

To introduce the topic of role play, I use this canned role-play demonstration to differentiate assertion from aggression. In this role play, I address a friend who habitually picks me up late to go to a meeting. A volunteer reads the canned lines in front of the group.

> *Friend:* Hi. Are you ready to go?
> *Response:* _____
> *Friend:* Oh, I hadn't noticed the time!
> *Response:* _____
> *Friend:* You're way too sensitive—I'm only fifteen minutes late!
> *Response:* _____
> *Friend:* Come on, you're being petty. What's the big deal?
> *Response:* _____
> *Friend:* You shouldn't feel that way!
> *Response:* _____
> *Friend:* I didn't realize it was important to you—I'll be on time next time.

Some of my sample responses to the canned lines are "You shouldn't tell me how I should feel" and "You're also much too sensitive" and "You're being petty, too!" Despite my lines being quite aggressive, filled with labeling, *you* statements, and a lot of tit-for-tat, because I am not yelling, most people, including audiences full of clinicians and other mental health professionals, think I am being assertive. Likewise, most people think that the person reading the canned lines was also assertive, and of course the lines are quite aggressive, filled with *You* statements, rhetorical questions, labeling, and put-downs. This shows the importance of *demonstrating* instead of *just talking about* assertiveness. Notice that the canned lines included the rhetorical question "What's the big deal?" Rhetorical questions are put-down statements disguised as questions.

It is surprising how many participants confuse assertiveness with aggressiveness, even when I explain the difference prior to the role play. This is one of the reasons I love role play in both individual and group sessions. So much more learning happens when people *experience* their learning firsthand instead of just talking about it.

In working with your clients, it is helpful to frequently refer to the main points to keep in mind—such as making sure the goal of your communication is to express yourself and not change someone else's mind or behavior. This helps clients stay focused and on track in developing their assertiveness skills.

☑ Mini-Lesson: Rhetorical Questions: Put-Downs Disguised as Questions

One of the most important lessons in the area of communication is identification of rhetorical questions. They are very common, but they are not really questions—they are judgmental put-downs. Angry exchanges are often filled with them, so it is beneficial to help your clients identify them.

Here are a few:

"What were you thinking?"
"Are you kidding me?"
"How many times do I need to remind you?"
"What's wrong with you?"
"Didn't I tell you that already?"
"Weren't you listening?"
"Why are you acting that way?"

Adding to the list is a fun brainstorming activity for your clients, both individually and in a group session. In a group situation, once a list is made, your clients can take turns being translators by interpreting the statement that is really being made, and then brainstorming rational alternatives. For example, in response to the rhetorical question, "What's wrong with you?" the translator volunteer could say, "You're an idiot."

Thus, the point of this exercise is to emphasize that rhetorical questions are really put-downs disguised as questions. After all, in response to "How many times do I need to remind you?" is there really an expectation that an actual number will be given in the answer?

This realization that rhetorical questions are really aggressive statements is a real eye opener for many clients. For clients who are "experts" at rhetorical questions, it helps them see that in dealing with difficult people, using their rhetorical questions actually makes them the difficult ones!

☑ DBT Technique: Practicing DEAR MAN

DBT is known for its experiential psychoeducational strategies, and the acronym DEAR MAN is one of the most commonly used change-based strategies of DBT for teaching assertive communication skills.

In DBT, acronyms serve as a guide for between-session practice, reminding clients of the specific communication skills needed, and as a guide in role-playing assertiveness strategies. Daily review and practice of skills learned in DBT group sessions is encouraged.

DEAR MAN

Describe the situation, non-judgmentally and objectively.

Express your thoughts and feelings tactfully.

Assert your wants and wishes clearly.

Reinforce others who respond positively by also being positive and expressing appreciation.

Mindful presence, without judgment, will help you be more open.

Accept the reactions of others rather than judging them! Do not raise your voice or talk in a way that demeans you.

Negotiate with others; compromise, instead of trying to get your way.

☑ Activity: Listing My Bill of Rights

Assertive communication is based on identifying personal rights. "Bill of Rights: Basic Human Rights and Corresponding Responsibilities" (Handout 6.6) has proved to be a great handout to give out after a group activity in which group participants brainstorm their personal rights.

I like to have people go around one by one and name a right that they have, such as the right to make a mistake, and then have them follow it with the corresponding responsibility. I am struck by how many clients—particularly women—are surprised that they have so many rights. Many of our clients, especially women, have been conditioned to be "nice" and "selfless" and learned early on not to make waves. In our society, it is more acceptable for men to show aggressive qualities, whereas women are rewarded for being more passive and "nice." Being raised in a family that rewards this double standard makes it even harder to overcome societal conditioning. The rewarding of women's self-denial and "selflessness," of course, leads to extremely low self-esteem and self-doubt. For these individuals, the Bill of Rights is a real eye-opener, and goes a long way toward improving their self-esteem and making their anxiety more manageable.

☑ Activity: Treat Others at Least as Good as an Egg!

A short and effective exercise for couple and family therapy, as well as for group sessions, is to use eggs to represent the fragility of relationships. Have on hand a few raw eggs (that you mark with a marker) and a few hard-boiled ones.

After telling your clients that some eggs are hard-boiled and some aren't (but without letting them know which ones are which), have them pass each egg from one person to another around the room. Not knowing which eggs are which, the clients will pass them all very slowly and gingerly. Make the point that even people who seem to be hard-boiled need to be handled gingerly and with care. All too often we don't handle our loved ones with care and softness, and we actually handle eggs better than the people in our lives.

To make more of an impact, identify the raw eggs (by the mark you made) and drop them on a plastic tarp as a demonstration that once an egg is cracked, you can't put it back together. This demonstrates that some relationships are cracked and cannot be put back together, so it is important not to take them for granted. A well-taken point is that if we are not careful with those close to us, feelings and relationships can be splattered, and just like Humpty Dumpty, they will never be the same. You can make other analogies with this visualization of eggs, as they are a great metaphor for human beings who have barriers and protective walls up on the outside, but are soft on the inside.

At one of my workplace wellness trainings, a participant walked out at the break saying, "I need to call my girlfriend and tell her I'm sorry." This shows that at heart, he really was a good egg!

☑ Activity: Turn Conflict Into a Win-Win

Another simple and quick exercise for couples, families, and groups is an activity that shows the importance of win-win solutions to conflict. All too often we think that for someone to win, someone else has to lose. This activity shows that the best solution is when everyone wins.

For this activity, two people stand facing each other without anything between them. Ask them to envision an imaginary line, and tell them that when you yell "Go!" they have 20 seconds to get their partner on their side.

After the exercise starts, there is usually a lot of playful pushing, pulling, bribing, and cajoling, although some partners realize that they both can win by simply switching sides—no drama involved.

When I work with couples in my office, I ask them to just switch sides (if they did not do so during the exercise) to show them how to have a "win-win." In a group situation, I have a pair who did it correctly demonstrate this win-win solution to the group. There is a lot of surprise accompanied by laughter when people see how they and their partner made things hard for themselves, when they both could have won without the cajoling and drama. The participants see how simple it all is once you have a win-win mentality!

☑ Activity: Nonverbal Communication Exercise

It's not what you say; it's *how* you say it! This very important lesson can be taught with this short, fun exercise. Use a phrase like "I never said he stole that watch" and have your client emphasize a different word each time:

I never said he stole that watch.
I *never* said he stole that watch.
I never *said* he stole that watch.
I never said *he* stole that watch.
I never said he *stole* that watch.
I never said he stole *that* watch.
I never said he stole that *watch.*

As you can quickly see, emphasizing a different word each time completely changes the meaning of the phrase each time. This is an excellent activity for helping your clients become more attuned to how things are said, not just the words that are spoken.

A Toolkit of Metaphors for Managing Conflict

Assembling a metaphorical relationship toolkit, with reminders about healthy communication and conflict resolution skills, is a fun activity for individuals, couples, and groups. Since relationships are crucial to our sense of well-being, most patients will benefit from visual reminders of the importance of staying assertive and building healthy relationships.

Toy soldier. Be strong and brave, even if life does not go your way. Identify your rights and fight for what you believe in! (Packages of toy soldiers can often be found at the dollar store.)

Toy firefighter. We should not be the one who starts the fire; rather, we should be the first to put it out! (These toy figures are also commonly found in dollars stores.)

Toy egg. Relationships are fragile. Treat those close to you at least as well as an egg! (Plastic Easter eggs work well for this exercise.)

Finger trap. If you and another person argue to prove you are right (that is, if you both pull), you will get stuck in the trap!

Miniature bowling pins. Don't let anyone else bowl you over! (Also found at the dollar store.)

Hershey Kisses and Hugs. Spread love and virtual kisses to others! Have a jar of these candies at work to spread the lovin' feeling, and make an effort to express positive thoughts and feelings to others. Remember to keep one for yourself to remind you that self-love is necessary before you can love anyone else.

Can you and your clients think of others?

Therapeutic Takeaways

☑ In helping your clients deal with difficult people, have them examine their communication to see if they are actually the difficult one.

☑ There are three types of communication: *assertive, nonassertive,* and *aggressive.* It is important for clients to learn what characterizes each one so they can identify these patterns in themselves and others.

☑ Assertive communication is healthy, rational, and respectful, whereas aggressive behavior is dominating and insensitive. Non-assertive communication results from insecurity and the need to be liked.

☑ Understanding and using role-play to incorporate interpersonal skills learning is crucial in developing assertiveness skills. Make sure your clients pay attention to the importance of the tone of voice, as it's not just *what* you say, but *how* you say it, that communicates the message.

☑ Using handouts as a resource while role-playing is vital in helping your clients improve their communication skills.

☑ Identifying basic human rights, along with corresponding responsibilities, helps people feel more comfortable with being assertive.

Handouts

The following worksheets will help your clients manage conflict. These handouts are all related to the lessons of this chapter. As a general guideline, handouts and assignments are given to your clients at the end of the session as homework, unless they are used in the session itself to illustrate points. Make sure you leave ample time to go over your expectations regarding the use of the selected handouts.

When assignments are given out, it is important to follow up with your clients at the beginning of the next session by reviewing and discussing their homework with them. Going over the homework is an essential aspect of being a solution-oriented therapist.

Note: All handouts in the book are available for download on my website by following the link below: http://www.belmontwellness.com/ultimate-solution-handouts/

Handout 6.1: Common Myths About Conflict

Myth 1: If someone is rude to you, it's okay if you call them on it and are rude back. Otherwise they will "get away with it."

Except when you need to protect your physical safety, it is never appropriate to be aggressive. By definition, aggression is being bossy and choosing for others instead of letting them choose for themselves. The goal of behavior is not healthy if it is to get your own way; it is healthier if your goal is to express your needs. (That doesn't mean you can't escalate the assertion, but the ability to meet your goal is not then contingent upon others' falling in line.) Express—don't impress!

Myth 2: If I start speaking assertively and it doesn't work, then it's okay to be aggressive.

The goal of assertiveness is not to get your way, but rather to ask for a change. Sometimes you don't get your way, but this doesn't justify getting aggressive. For example, it is hard for some parents not to get bossy when their child doesn't listen, but setting limits and consequences—rather than being bossy—is much more respectful to children and pays off in the long run.

Myth 3: There are situations in which it is best to be non-assertive.

By definition, non-assertive behavior is self-denying, people pleasing, and motivated by fear and insecurity. It is never desirable to have low self-esteem and people-pleasing neediness. However, there are times when you might decide—after weighing the pros and cons—not to assert yourself. This assertive decision comes from a place of confidence. You decide out of logic, not fear. The rational decision to not assert yourself is still an assertive one!

For example, if you only see your Uncle Harry once a year, you might not want to assert yourself by telling him that he has bad body odor. However, if you see him daily or even weekly, or if he lives with you, then you might decide to say something!

Myth 4: People who are aggressive (bullies) are very confident in themselves.

Certainly this type of communicator seems to feel superior and righteous, but the reasons behind bullies' behavior are faulty thinking, negativity, and insecurity. People who are aggressive are generally not happy campers, and their show of strength hides a lot of weakness and vulnerability. Also, many people remain nonassertive for too long and then eventually blow up.

Myth 5: People who learn the differences among the three types of communication can readily apply them.

It's one thing to recognize the differences among the three types of communication and to be able to identify them. Old habits are hard to break, and the communication style people develop is part of their personality which has been adaptive over time in response to their unique situation. It might look easy to change your communication style, but this can be quite challenging for those who haven't really learned how to express themselves confidently, and who do not feel confident inside. It takes a lot of practice to change the thinking patterns that lie beneath unhealthy communication. It is like learning a new language—often the accent is hard to break!

Handout 6.2: The Three Types of Communication

Characteristics		
Nonassertive Behavior	**Assertive Behavior**	**Aggressive Behavior**
• Inhibited • Lets others violate rights • Does not stand up for rights • Afraid of "making waves" • Lets others choose • Unconfident, nervous	• "I" statements • Expresses and asserts own rights, needs, desires • Stands up for legitimate rights without violating rights of others • Emotionally honest, direct, expressive	• "You" statements • Expresses own rights at expense of others • Has inappropriate outbursts or hostile overreactions • Emotionally honest and direct at others' expense
Feelings That Result		
• Hurt, anxious, disappointed in self at the time and possibly angry later	• Confident, self-respecting; feels good about self and others	• Angry, then righteous; superior, resentful, possibly guilty later
Effects		
• Individual avoids unpleasant and risky situations, conflict • Individual feels "used," accumulates anger, feels nonvalued	• Individual feels good, validated by self and others • Individual experiences improved self-confidence, gets needs met; relationships are freer and more honest	• Saved-up anger "justifies" a blowup • Individual has emotional outbursts "to get even"

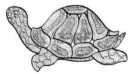

Nonassertive behavior is being like a turtle: hiding and being protective to be on the "safe" side, avoidant

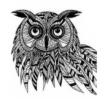

Assertive communication is being like a wise owl: thinking rationally, standing upright, being confident, and showing wisdom without impulsivity

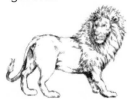

Aggressive behavior is represented by a lion: powerful, mighty, strong, threatening, while violating the rights of others

Handout 6.3: Comparing the Three Types of Communication

Nonassertive Behavior	Assertive Behavior	Aggressive Behavior
Keeps things in; doesn't speak up	Uses "I" statements	Uses "You" statements
Suppresses own rights and needs	Asserts own rights, needs, desires	Expresses own rights at expense of others
Denies need to make others like him/her or approve	Tries to get needs met while not violating rights of others	Gets needs met, but at others' expense; puts others down in the process
Permits others to infringe on his/her rights	Sets limits and priorities	Violates rights of others
Emotionally dishonest, indirect, inhibited, approval seeking	Confident, calm, secure	Honest without tact; bluntly direct; self-righteous
Self-denying	Chooses for self	Chooses for others
Emotional Costs of Nonassertion	*Emotional Benefits of Assertion*	*Emotional Costs of Aggression*
Feels hurt, anxious, afraid of others' reactions	Is confident, self-respecting; feels good about self	Feels angry, indignant, righteous
Self-blame	Self-affirmation	Blame, criticism, and judgment of others
Payoffs of Nonassertion	*Payoffs of Assertion*	*Payoffs of Aggression*
Does not "make waves"; avoids conflict	Relationships are open and honest	Feels as if justice has been served; feels superior to others
Shies away from taking risks	Feels satisfied about expressing self	Keeps others at a distance
Is people pleasing; avoids having others gets mad at him/her	Not obligated by what people think	Might get his/her own way, despite infringing on others' rights

Handout 6.4: Turn *You* Statements Into *I* Statements

The basis of this activity is shown in Handout 6.4. This worksheet will give you practice turning "You" messages into "I" messages.

"You" statements are a characteristic of aggressive communication, while "I" statements are a characteristic of assertive communication. "You" statements are judgmental towards others, while "I" statements are less judgmental and more descriptive, allowing you to stick to the facts and not interpretations.

Examples of "You" Statements:

"You are being so rude."
"You should know better."
"You make me so upset!"
"It's none of your business!"

Examples of "I" Statements:

"I feel uncomfortable when you raise your voice at me."
"I thought you had known that."
"I was upset when you said that."
"I don't feel comfortable discussing personal issues."

For the following examples, turn "You" statements into "I" statements.

"You" Statements	"I" Statements
"You make me so mad!"	_____
"You never listen to me!"	_____
"You're too sensitive!"	_____

Now it's your turn to think of your own examples from your own life, changing "you" statements to "I" statements.

"You" Statements	"I" Statements
_____	_____
_____	_____
_____	_____
_____	_____
_____	_____

Handout 6.5: Aggressive Behavior:
Reasons, Payoffs, and Consequences

REASONS

1. *Confusion between a feeling and an action.* It is often not understood that anger is a feeling and aggression is a behavior. Feelings are acceptable, but aggressive behavior is not.
2. *Prior non-assertion.* Anger builds up, you feel that your rights have been violated too many times, and you feel righteous and indignant. Hurt and tension explodes.
3. *Sense of superiority and self-righteousness.* You feel that you are standing up for what is right, and that aggression is justified.
4. *Need to control and dominate.* You feel that by controlling the other person, you can get your way and make things right. Your motto is "Attack before you are attacked."
5. *Overreaction due to past emotional experiences.* Unresolved emotions are inappropriately played out in present situations.
6. *Mistaken view of aggression as desirable.* You believe that aggression is the best way to get your needs met, make things right, and get people to act the way you want them to.
7. *Skills deficit.* You have not learned ways to manage your anger, possess low frustration tolerance, and don't know how to control your impulses.

PAYOFFS

1. Aggression lets off steam; it's easier in the short run to "let it out."
2. Aggression feels superior and righteous.
3. Aggression seems to show that you are strong, hiding your weakness and vulnerability.
4. Aggression gets your needs met, your way.
5. Aggression allows you to blame others so you don't have to take responsibility for your behavior.

CONSEQUENCES

1. Aggression alienates others, and then leaves you feeling isolated.
2. Aggression often leads to your feeling guilty later.
3. Aggression leads to conflict-ridden relationships.
4. Aggression keeps you harboring negativity and resentment.

Handout 6.6: Bill of Rights: Basic Human Rights and Corresponding Responsibilities

I have the right:	*I have the responsibility:*
To be treated fairly	To treat others fairly
To express feelings, including anger	To accept the feelings of others
To change my mind	To accept others' changing their minds
To make mistakes	To admit my mistakes
To ask for help	To offer help to others
To not be perfect	To not expect perfection in others
To be honest	To be tactful
To set limits and priorities	To respect the limits of others
To forgive myself	To forgive others
To end relationships that are unhealthy	To give feedback about why
To make my own decisions	To accept the consequences
To say "no" and not feel guilty	To accept "no" from others
To change	To support growth in others
To make my own decisions	To not decide for others
To expect respect	To set limits on disrespectful behavior
To fail	To try my best
To not please everybody	To please myself

The Conflict Solution

Handout 6.7: Communication Basics

Assertive Communication Enhancers	Aggressive Communication Stoppers
I don't agree with you.	That's ridiculous!
I don't think that it will work.	That will never work!
I do not think you understand.	You're not listening to me!
I don't think that it's practical.	It's just not practical!
I'd be surprised if that happened.	It's impossible.
I feel like you ignore me often.	You're never available!
That happens quite often.	That always happens!

Aggressive Responses	Assertive Responses
Characterized by "You" statements	*Characterized by "I" statements*
Goal is to change others	*Goal is to ask for a change*
Goal is to IMPRESS	*Goal is to EXPRESS*
Goal is to PROVE	*Goal is to IMPROVE*
Violate others' rights	*Stand up for others' rights*
Bossy	*Respectful*
Honest, but tactless	*Emotionally honest, but tactful*
Get even, seek revenge	*No "tit for tat"*

REMEMBER!!!!!!

- Use "I" statements.
- Don't over-explain or over-apologize.
- Don't get sidetracked.
- Keep your goal in mind.
- Focus on the behavior, not the person.
- Describe; don't judge or evaluate.
- Another's aggression does not justify counteraggression.
- Someone else does not need to set the tone for your own behavior.
- Be generous with sincere praise and positive feedback.

Handout 6.8: Checklist for Assertive Communication

This checklist is a great reminder to use when you coach your clients on how to be more assertive and will help you structure your role plays with individual and group clients.

1. Ask yourself, "What is my goal?" Make sure it is an assertive goal.
2. Use "I" statements.
3. Strive to express, not impress!
4. Use reasons, not excuses—don't over-explain or over-apologize.
5. Be in control, not controlling!
6. No "shoulding" on yourself or others!
7. Avoid rhetorical questions, which are put-downs disguised as questions.
8. Think rationally—separate your perceptions from the facts.
9. Use good listening skills—don't just hear!
10. Use assertive nonverbals to match your assertive verbals.
11. Avoid the need to be right.
12. Identify your personal rights and corresponding responsibilities.
13. Weigh the pros and cons of being assertive—decide if you want to assert yourself!
14. Show empathy and acceptance of the other person.
15. Practice your assertive skills and ask for feedback.

. . . AND REMEMBER!!!!!!

✓ Don't get sidetracked; always keep your goal in mind.
✓ Do not label others or be judgmental—rather, be descriptive.
✓ Another's aggression does not justify counteraggression.
✓ Don't let someone else's negativity set the tone for your own behavior.
✓ Remember your sense of humor!

Handout 6.9: My Communication Diary

Examples of Assertive Communication	My Goal and Outcome My Healthy Thoughts
Examples of Aggressive Communication	My Goal and Outcome My Unhealthy Thoughts Alternative Responses
Examples of Non-Assertive Communication	My Goal and Outcome My Unhealthy Thoughts Alternative Responses
Communication Style Benefits	Communication Style Costs
My Conclusions and Plan for Improving My Communication	

Handout 6.10: My Communication-Tracking Log

Weekly Assertiveness Log

Date(s): _____

1. My general communication style

_____

2. My emotional responses

_____

3. Degree of negative feelings   LOW 1 2 3 4 5 6 7 8 9 10 HIGH

4. Unhealthy thoughts

_____

    Certainty of beliefs   LOW 1 2 3 4 5 6 7 8 9 10 HIGH

5. Healthy thoughts

_____

    Certainty of beliefs   LOW 1 2 3 4 5 6 7 8 9 10 HIGH

6. Communication skills I have practiced

_____

7. Steps I have taken to be more assertive

_____

8. Alternative skills I can use to be assertive

_____

9. Costs and benefits of my communication style

_____

10. Goals for improving my communication

_____

Recommended Resources

Self-Help Books

Your Perfect Right: Assertiveness and Equality in Your Life and Relationships
Robert Alberti and Michael Emmons

The New Assertive Woman: Be Your Own Person Through Assertive Training
Lynn Z. Bloom, Karen Coburn, and Joan Perlman

The Messages Workbook: Powerful Strategies for Effective Communication at Work & Home
Martha Davis, Kim Paleg, and Patrick Fanning

How to Communicate: The Ultimate Guide to Improving Your Personal and Professional Relationships
Matthew McKay, Martha Davis, and Patrick Fanning

Clinician Books

A Manual for Assertiveness Trainers (Volume II of the Professional Edition: Your Perfect Right)
Robert E. Alberti and Michael L. Emmons

86 TIPS (Treatment Ideas & Practical Strategies) for the Therapeutic Toolbox
Judith A. Belmont

103 Group Activities and TIPS (Treatment Ideas & Practical Strategies)
Judith A. Belmont

127 More Amazing Tips and Tools for the Therapeutic Toolbox
Judith A. Belmont

Responsible Assertive Behavior: Cognitive/Behavioral Procedures for Trainers
Arthur J. Lange and Patricia Jakubowski

Messages: The Communication Skills Book
Matthew McKay, Martha Davis, and Patrick Fanning

Links

Mind Tools

"Communication Skills"

www.mindtools.com/page8.html

Psychology Tools

(Assertiveness worksheets)

http://www.psychologytools.org/assertiveness.html

Therapist Aid

(Assertiveness worksheets)

http://www.therapistaid.com/therapy-worksheets/none/none

WikiHow

"How to Be Assertive"

http://www.wikihow.com/Be-Assertive

CHAPTER SEVEN

The Forgiveness Solution
Helping Your Clients Set Themselves Free

With the emergence of Positive Psychology, common issues that affect every human being, such as life satisfaction, happiness, wellness, gratitude, and forgiveness, have become a focus of mainstream psychological practice. Forgiveness is an essential act that determines not only our state of mind but also our relationships with others. Since we live in a world with flawed humans just like us, there is no shortage of reasons for every human to be angry, hold grudges, and feel wronged. From an ex-spouse who we think has made our life miserable, to parents who did not treat us the way we deserved, to coworkers, friends and classmates who treated us disrespectfully or even betrayed us, to our children who did not turn out the way we raised them to be despite all the good lessons and opportunities we gave them, the people in our lives do things that often seems unforgivable. As clinicians, we often find ourselves helping our clients through the healing process of forgiveness. To add further complexity to this picture, it is not uncommon for our clients to come to therapy because the ones they find it hardest to forgive are themselves. Guilt for not having the foresight to know what they know now in hindsight weighs heavily on those who feel as if they have somehow caused damage to themselves or others in their lives when all they wanted was to be *helpful* and *good*. I have had many clients who felt ashamed and think of themselves as *bad* when important relationships in their lives did not turn out the way they wanted them to, and they take more than their share of responsibility when people and events in their lives go awry, leading to self-blame and disappointment in oneself and in life.

The degree to which our clients are able to forgive either themselves or others is the degree to which they will be able to live with a self-confident, healthy and optimistic attitude. Part of the reason for this is that a lack of forgiveness is an expression of pain and bitterness at having been *wrong* or having been *wronged*—or at least at *perceiving* that one was *wrong* or has been *wronged*. In a world where there are many shades of gray, people who are stuck in blame are stuck in black-and-white thinking. The hurt our clients experience when they feel slighted and ignored—or worse yet, rebuffed—goes deep to the core of their sense of life injustice. Despite knowing that life is not fair, our clients still often expect it to be, and become indignant when it isn't. When our clients struggle with being able to forgive, the work of therapy is a journey in exploring pain, the grievance story behind the pain, and how to find the courage to heal through forgiveness. At times, my clients question whether they really have to forgive to move on. I tell them, only if they want to stop defining themselves by moments in the past.

Forgiveness is not just a psychological concept that is good for the head. Studies have shown that it is good for the body and physical health, and can even extend one's life. Along with good nutrition with plenty of fruits and vegetables, exercise, and maintaining a healthy weight, the ability to forgive seems to correlate with a healthier and longer life. Researchers have found that the ability to forgive is actually good for one's heart, both figuratively and literally. Lawler and her fellow researchers at East Carolina University found that forgiveness improved quality of sleep and lowered blood pressure and heart rate (Lawler et al., 2003, 2005). Conversely, they found that holding on to resentments correlated with insomnia. In another study, Touissant, Owen, and Cheadle (2012) discovered a correlation between forgiveness and lower mortality rates due to healthier functioning of the cardiovascular and endocrine systems. In their 2012 study published in the Journal of Behavioral Medicine using a poll of 1,500 U.S. citizens over the age of 66, those who agreed with the statement "Before I can forgive others, they must apologize to me for the things they have done" or "Before I can forgive others, they must promise not to do the same thing again" were more likely to die within three years than those who did not agree with those statements (Toussaint et al, 2012).

Terrie Heinrich Rizzo, manager of health and fitness education programs for the Stanford University Health Improvement Program and executive director of Personally Fit Belgium, refers to forgiveness as "A Hot Field in Clinical Psychology" (Rizzio, 2006). She reports that back in 1997 there were only 58 studies on the effects of forgiveness, as compared to 1,200 published studies just a decade later pointing to the mind-body effects of forgiveness. In summary, she stated that the study of forgiveness is part of a fundamental shift to a more positive and less disease-focused orientation of psychological study. She noted that one of the common themes in these studies is that forgiveness alleviates stress, thereby lessening negative physiological reactions such as increased blood pressure, higher adrenaline, immune suppression, and impaired neurological functioning. She also noted that those who were forgiving tended to have stronger social networks, which also correlates with improved physical as well as psychological health.

Even leading research health institutions such as the Mayo Clinic emphasize the healing power of forgiveness. On Mayo's public website, readers are educated on the importance of healing through the power of forgiveness (Mayo Clinic Staff, 2011). Among some of the health benefits already mentioned in this section, they cite the correlation of forgiveness with fewer symptoms of depression, anxiety, and substance abuse, along with increased spiritual and psychological well-being.

Before working with your clients on forgiving themselves or others, they will likely need some education on what forgiveness means and what it does not mean. Judging from my clients' common misperceptions, forgiveness appears to be one of the most misunderstood human acts. So many clients struggle with this topic, and until they dispel some of the common myths of what forgiveness means, they remain stuck in the land of blame, grudges, hurt, and anger. All too often my clients have waited for the offending parties to say they were sorry before forgiving, and have not realized that you can forgive even if they are not sorry. After all, once my clients learn that forgiveness is a gift they give to themselves because they (the clients) deserve it even if the transgressor does not, they are freeing themselves from moments in the past. It does not mean they condone the behavior; it just means they don't want to be imprisoned by what happened anymore.

In the following section, I have highlighted some techniques to help people forgive. First and foremost, however, some psychoeducational mini-lessons are essential for combating the myths and misperceptions of what forgiveness is. One of my major points in this section is that the process of forgiveness can be compared to the process of grieving and healing from loss. Thus, in the treatment tips section, I offer ideas on how to educate your clients about forgiveness, including how to educate them on using Kubler-Ross's five-stages-of-grieving model to help them heal from hurt and loss, which is essential to moving on to forgiveness.

Treatment Tips

☑ Mini-Lesson: Clarify Truths and Realities of Forgiveness

Forgiveness is one of the most misunderstood concepts that we deal with in helping clients move on from past hurts inflicted by others. Below are five tips for helping your clients learn what forgiveness is and what it is not. Often, even if clients logically agree with the points made in this section, the may not yet have a deep acceptance of these principles. "Common Myths About Forgiveness" (Handout 7.1) offers a good foundation for a discussion on what forgiveness is, and is a good handout for your clients to read as homework to begin their work on forgiveness.

"Healing Thoughts for Forgiveness" (Handout 7.2) can also offer your clients some insight into the ways they can change their thinking to heal and forgive. "Quick Test: What Is Your Forgiveness IQ?" (Handout 7.6) can be a fun and informative way to help your clients identify and remember 10 important ingredients to forgiveness.

TIP 1: FORGIVENESS IS NOT SAYING IT'S OKAY.
Forgiveness is often misunderstood as letting someone off the hook or condoning behavior that is hurtful or wrong. This couldn't be further

from the truth. You can share with your clients that even if others don't deserve their forgiveness, they deserve to forgive. It is they who deserve not to hold on to negativity and bitterness, because it holds them back in the past. Forgiveness is more about letting go of the hurt and not being a victim anymore, and transforming your role from that of a victim to that of a survivor.

Furthermore, the idea that someone needs to be sorry to be forgiven will keep your clients stuck waiting for people to change. Some people won't change, but by emphasizing to our clients that the only people that they can change are themselves is enormously empowering. When your clients learn that the people in their lives that have wronged them don't have to be sorry in order to be forgiven, they can reframe their blame in a whole new light. When clients realize that forgiveness is so much more about themselves than it is about the transgressors, they feel much better about choosing the path of forgiveness.

TIP 2: BEING UNFORGIVING IMPAIRS YOUR HEALTH.
Various studies have shown that bearing a grudge and being unforgiving can shorten your life. Forgiveness expert Fred Luskin from the Stanford Forgiveness Project claims that "holding a grudge is hazardous to your health" (Luskin, 2003). He is referring not only to mental and emotional health, but also to physical health. He emphasizes in his writings that bitterness and hostility that people harbor are correlated with heart disease and stroke, and cause individuals to live shorter lives than their less angry counterparts.

TIP 3: FORGIVENESS IS A TRAINABLE SKILL.
Forgiveness might not come naturally to many of our clients. Finding out that it is a skill that they can learn is very enlightening and also very comforting. Therapists can offer clients some concrete steps to forgiveness. In his Stanford forgiveness project, Luskin (2003) offers a summary of nine steps. These pointers taken from his nine step blueprint can offer some good guidelines for you and your client when working on the forgiveness

1. Tell at least one or two people about your hurt. Healing is more likely when you share it with others.
2. Make a choice to forgive. Identify what happened, be clear about why you have a grievance, and make it a choice to forgive anyway.
3. Distance yourself from the hurt by taking the life experience less personally.
4. Keep the hurt in perspective, acknowledging that hurt from the past is being kept alive from the thoughts of the upset. Focus on the feelings and thoughts that result from the hurt rather than the acts of the past.
5. Practice stress management techniques to relax and soothe.
6. Let go of the expectation that people can give you what they do not have to give, and adopt the perspective that there is hope for a better life without expecting them to change.
7. Build on the experience and make something positive out of the hurt.
8. Take your personal power back by focusing on love and beauty in the present moment.
9. Have your grievance story remind you to be forgiving and to see this as a heroic choice.

TIP 4: FORGIVENESS DOES NOT MEAN YOU GO BACK FOR MORE.

Just because you forgive, it doesn't mean that you even maintain a relationship with the people who have wronged you. You can forgive them for being too unhealthy for you to continue a relationship with them, while also forgiving them for being too impaired to change. Protecting yourself and not allowing yourself to be hurt anymore comes from a position of mental clarity and identification of your right not to be mistreated.

When you make the decision to distance yourself from toxic people in your life, however, sometimes you will not be able to distance yourself completely. Consider the case of dealing with a close family member, such as an adult child. In these cases, setting firm limits and boundaries and not enabling disrespectful behavior becomes the goal in treatment.

Tip 5: Self-forgiveness is essential to a healthy and positive life.

Perhaps the people that our clients have the most difficulty forgiving are themselves. Judging yourself for not being the perfect student, worker, parent, child, spouse, friend, and so forth is a sentence that people impose on themselves. Some amount of remorse and guilt is of course normal in living a responsible life, but all too often our clients are too harsh with themselves for their past mistakes, which end up defining them and limiting their ability to move on. Helping your clients have self-compassion is essential to the healing process.

The best way for clients to move on from their mistakes is to learn from them and use better judgment now. They won't be perfect, but when they are assured that they are a work in progress, they can learn to be easier on themselves. After all, we always have a chance to improve on yesterday, no matter where we are in life.

Tip 6: Forgiveness is a choice

Forgiveness doesn't usually just happen—you have to choose it. Once your clients realize that forgiveness is a gift to themselves, and maybe to the other person secondarily, they may have an easier time making the choice to forgive. Some clients still can't part with their sense of having been wronged, but these clients pay for that rigidity immensely, as if they swallowed a bitter pill. The clients that have the best chance to reinvent themselves as they age are those who allow themselves to let go of bitterness and slights. This does not mean that the hurt and the scars aren't still there, but they are no longer figuratively picked at and allowed to fester.

☑ Mini-Lesson: Kubler-Ross's Five Stages of Grieving

After educating your client on what forgiveness is and what it is not, clarifying any common misunderstandings, the next step is to help them heal from their memories. When my clients are struggling with forgiveness, I offer the model of the five stages of grieving (Kubler-Ross, 1969). When we think of grieving, we think of dealing with a physical death, whether that be facing your own mortality or the death of a loved one. But as we learn in Judith Viorst's *Necessary Losses* (1986), loss is also about death of a dream, death of a relationship, the loss of "impossible expectations," a death of our innocence and trust. In order for us to have new beginnings in life, we can't be hanging on too much to the old losses, as then we won't have room for opening our hearts to new possibilities.

Lily Tomlin once said, "Forgiveness means giving up all hope for a better past." This very poignant quote points to the importance of seeing forgiveness as part of a grieving process to let go of the past, putting to rest what should have been or could have been but never was. Linda, a 38-year-old mother of three, is an example of a client who found herself imprisoned by her inability to forgive. As the child of a controlling and very critical, anxious mother and a verbally abusive father, Linda found that much of her adult life was spent in a state of low-grade sadness mixed with anger. With her family as well as with people at work, she frequently found triggers that ended up reverberating back to past themes from her family of origin. Any hint of reference to her not being good enough or any feeling that she was being criticized would sink her into a funk, followed by indignation at others' rudeness and untrustworthiness. She constantly sought approval from others but never felt as if she ever really got it. Twenty years after being told in her youth that she was not smart, that she was selfish, and that she was a "whore," she still believed these labels and felt bad and dirty, even though she had been faithfully married for 13 years and was very giving to her husband, children, and friends.

Even in therapy, Linda was constantly afraid of being annoying to me, and apologized profusely if she felt as if she was repeating the same problems over and over again. Even though I told her that clients are supposed to have problems—that's why they come to therapy, and otherwise I wouldn't have a job—she still felt like a burden. She felt as if at some point I would be done hearing her same stuff over and over again. In fear of being rejected, as she had been by her parents, she toyed frequently with the idea of stopping her sessions—basically, rejecting me before I rejected her. This continued for years. Her fear of being annoying to me was so strong because she was so annoyed at herself, stemming from her sense that her parents were always so annoyed with her.

Even though Linda had distanced herself from her parents physically; had only very occasional, brief phone calls with them; and had not seen them in years despite living just a few hours away, she kept their conversation and the relationship alive and well in her head. Their critical messages remained on "life support," although she kept hoping that the physical limit setting would allow her to erect a metaphorical fence in her head and keep them out. For years in therapy, she remained stuck in her shame and blame of her parents for their emotional and verbal abuse. It was all very intertwined.

Linda was steadfast in maintaining that her parents did not deserve to be "let off the hook" and that she could never forgive them for treating her the way they did. She carried so much anger and hurt inside, and refused to soften her stance for quite some time in treatment since she did not think that they *deserved it.* She thought that forgiveness means that you are condoning bad behavior, and she refused to condone what had happened to her. Despite the fact that I tried to teach her otherwise, she would not give up the grudge. She felt as if that was the key to keeping her parents out of her life, but in fact it gave them more room inside her head and actually locked them in there with her rigid attitude—inside the virtual fence she had erected to keep them out.

The turning point in therapy came when Linda finally had the courage to work on forgiving her parents. She had fought it for so long, but luckily she lost the fight, because that was a fight she could never win. After being in so much pain and self-doubt, she eventually developed enough trust in our relationship that she accepted my suggestion that she forgive them on the basis of them being emotionally sick and mentally ill people who did not know any better. After all, people can only give you what they have to give, and they didn't have the mental health to give her the love and security they didn't have themselves. I used handouts such as "The Five Stages of Grieving and Healing" (Handout 7.5), based on Kubler-Ross's model (1969). As you can see, on the left-hand side are thoughts relevant to the actual grieving of the death of a loved one, and on the right-hand side are the thoughts accompanying healing from a trauma, loss, disappointment, or unfulfilled dream. I have long used Kubler-Ross's stages of death and dying to symbolize healing from a memory or a major life disappointment. Linda grieved the loss of the parents that she would never have, and finally reached a point where she could move past the anger to a state of acceptance, the final stage of the model. Only then could she grow from the hurt instead of being held back by it. Only by forgiving them could she start trusting others more in her life, including her spouse.

Knowledge of what forgiveness is, and going through the stages of grieving, were what Linda needed to move on from her pain and give herself the gift of forgiveness.

☑ Mini-Lesson: The Four Things That Matter Most

As previously emphasized, bibliotherapy is an important part of solution-oriented therapy. This could not be truer than in the area of forgiveness. Because this topic touches so many emotional chords and past hurts, bibliotherapy with well-selected books can offer opportunities for between-session processing and healing. Ira Byock's *The Four Things That Matter Most* (2004), is one book that I recommend to clients struggling with a need to forgive or a need to be forgiven because of their own past behaviors that they now regret. Byock, a palliative care physician, describes the four phrases that are relevant for the living as well as for the dying. From his 30 plus years of being a physician, he has boiled down what matters most to four sentiments:

Please forgive me
I forgive you
I thank you
I love you

In his book, Byock offers examples of patients who have been wronged and have themselves wronged others, and how they have dealt with those close to them in the stages of dying. He gives the example of a middle-aged man whose abusive, neglectful, and now estranged father was dying. Despite what he had gone through at the hands of his dad, when he approached his dying father in the hospital room, he requested of him to "please forgive me." He acknowledged to his father that he must have had his own pain that prompted him to treat him like he did—he must have been disappointed at his not being the son he wanted. The next part of the conversation was "I forgive you." After that, the son thanked his dad for the lessons learned, and lastly said, "I love you." Byock urges us to ask for forgiveness first, and from there it is easier to mutually forgive. He acknowledges that people who do bad things are in pain, too. In his book, Byock recommends having this conversation even with a deceased parent through a letter, journaling, or just having the conversation in your head. To quote playwright Robert Anderson in his play *I Never Sang for My Father*, "Death ends a life, but it does not end a relationship."

Byock's book is a great one to recommend to clients who are struggling with issues of forgiveness, and for some it may unlock the keys to healing.

After offering your clients psychoeducation regarding forgiveness and encouraging them to heal, the next step is to offer practical, hands-on strategies to help your clients forgive.

☑ Activity: Using Metaphors and Visualizations

Once your clients have more understanding of what forgiveness is and is not, the next step is to use metaphors and visualizations to unlock their ability to forgive.

The use of metaphors is a common tool for in Cognitive Behavior Therapy (CBT) as well as in Dialectical Behavior Therapy (DBT), Acceptance and Commitment Therapy (ACT), and other third-wave approaches. Metaphors are increasingly being used in modern treatment approaches, capitalizing on the power and impact that they offer. Metaphors are invaluable tools for helping clients get "unstuck" from old habits of thinking by providing a refreshing away to look at things.

Images and metaphorical stories make it easier to recall important ideas. Lyddon, Clay, and Sparks (2001) offer reasons why metaphors are so important in treatment: They help clients establish rapport, they help clients access their emotions in a nonthreatening way, and they help clients think in new and creative ways.

Forgiveness is an especially great area to use metaphors. For deep-seated wounds, emotional imagery is effective in helping clients let go of grudges and hurts. There are some hurts so deep that words and thoughts alone don't have enough healing power.

Following are metaphors that I suggest using to help your clients in the process of forgiveness. The opportunity to use metaphor is limitless—and the following ideas might trigger you to think of some of your own to use with clients:

1. ACT founder Steven Hayes uses the image of a hook for demonstrating a lack of forgiveness. The person stuck in a lack of forgiveness as well as the transgressor are both on a hook, and only by getting the transgressor off first can the other get off the hook too.

2. Another popular ACT metaphor that can be applied to the topic of forgiveness is quicksand. The more we fight and try to get out of the quicksand, the deeper we sink. However, by stopping the struggle and ceasing to resist it by lying flat, we will be able to stay on top of the quicksand. Although Hayes's point with this metaphor is that the more we fight against feeling pain and suffering, the more we suffer, the same lesson can be applied to the topic of forgiveness. The more we fight the choice to forgive, the more we sink in deeper in bitterness and pain.

3. Forgiveness is like immersing yourself in an ocean, cleansing yourself of the hurt.

4. Forgiveness is like taking off a backpack filled with resentments and grudges. The more you take off, the lighter your load will be.

5. Life support is another great metaphor. We keep resentments alive by not pulling the plug.

6. The ACT metaphor of a beach ball in a body of water is a powerful one to relate to forgiveness. Resistance to forgiveness is like trying to push an inflated beach ball under the water—it keeps on popping back up!

☑ Activity: Forgiveness and Gratitude Lists

Spiritual writer Doreen Virtue (1998) suggests having your clients make a list of all the people in their past who have hurt them. The list can include people who your clients have already forgiven, not necessarily the ones your clients are focusing on now.

In session, have your clients go over their list, reading the names and describing to you one at a time why the acts were hurtful. In a group situation, you can have each person share one example with the group. As your clients describe each situation, encourage them to visualize the person and to say words of forgiveness to each person. Have them name the transgression that they are forgiving the person for. Virtue suggests ending each example with words such as, "I forgive you totally and completely. I release you and I release me. We are both now free."

Another type of list to suggest to your clients is a gratitude list. Ask your clients to think of people they have trouble forgiving. Beside the list of hurts, have them write the gifts they have received by growing through the hurt. This idea reflects Byock's focus (2004) for the third thing that matters that he address in his book, *The Four Things That Matter Most*, which is the ability to express gratefulness in saying "Thank you." It might seem like a stretch for clients to actually be grateful to their perpetrators, but in recognizing the healing power of forgiveness and realizing the gifts they have learned from their challenges, they might find they have the strength to "deepen and not weaken."

☑ Activity: Journaling and Log-Keeping for Forgiveness

Many forgiveness exercises involve some type of writing. Writing helps to get thoughts out, putting them *out there* and out of your head. Some events in our life are so hurtful that only by getting them out on paper are we able to let them loosen their hold on us. Thus, writing helps your clients be more objective and put their hurts in perspective.

"Healing Thoughts for Forgiveness" (Handout 7.2) can be a helpful handout to use as a basis for thinking about topics to include and address in forgiveness journaling. For clients who want or need more structure, "Journaling for Forgiveness" (Handout 7.4) offers a worksheet for processing feelings and thoughts. You might also want to offer them the "Weekly Forgiveness Log" (Handout 7.7) to accompany their journaling. This handout offers a way for clients to summarize the work they have been doing in session. "My Forgiveness Log" (Handout 7.3) provides another tool to help clients clarify their thoughts, feelings, and behaviors, with an emphasis on having them rate the degree of conviction they have for their thoughts.

For another assignment, you might suggest to your clients that each week they pick one person to work on forgiving, fill out one of the handouts or compose a journal entry about that person, and then go over it in session.

Here are some elements you can suggest that your clients include in a journal entry:

What happened
How it hurt before
How it still hurts
How this hurt has held them back
How the hurt has helped them grow
Strategies they are using to heal
Visualizations and metaphors that help them heal
Behavioral steps or goals for letting go of the hurt and anger

☑ Activity: Write a Forgiveness Letter

Writing a letter to someone who has hurt you can be very powerful. These letters are usually not sent, and if they are, they need to be conciliatory and not inflammatory!

Writing letters without the expectation of sending them allows your clients the opportunity to express their grievances. My clients have often asked me why they should bother, as they don't plan to send it anyway, and besides, sometimes the people they are most angry at are no longer alive. I respond that healing does not have to involve the other person; in fact, at times that just complicates matters. Since forgiveness is something clients do for themselves, just the act of expressing themselves can be healing.

I have had my clients write letters to, for example, parents who are no longer living. At first the letters are generally angry letters—"letting them have it." After that is processed, I ask my clients to write a second letter with the wisdom they have now, with the understanding that although the behaviors were bad, these people were not really bad— just unhealthy. After all, people can only act as healthy as they are, and people cannot give you what they do not have to give. Writing a letter from this stance can be healing once the anger is expressed in the initial letter.

These letter-writing exercises often bring up a lot of pain in my clients, as they still have very raw hurt from what happened to them; to conjure it up again is difficult. I assure them that opening up the wound is better than not allowing it to heal—sometimes you need to take off the Band-Aid. It hurts when it is pulled off, but the fresh air and cleaning does the wound good. The wound can then be dressed and bandaged again, but this time it will likely stay cleaner than before.

In the case of self-forgiveness, I have had clients write letters to their earlier selves that did not know any better. In this activity, clients write a letter to themselves, explaining why they cannot forgive themselves. They then follow it up with a letter that uses a more objective approach, using cognitive challenges to their assumptions, perhaps using the costive distortion list from "My Daily Thought Log" (Handout 3.3).

At the end of the letter, clients may want to release the person from having a hold on them anymore. Then they can either burn the printed paper, rip the letter into little pieces, or have some "ceremony" where they release the letter and everything written on it.

☑ CBT Technique: Cost/Benefit Analysis for Forgiveness

The popular CBT approach of performing a cost/benefit analysis is also very powerful in helping your clients work on their ability to forgive. In this approach, clients are instructed to divide a piece of paper into two columns: the costs of forgiving on one side and the benefits of forgiving on the other side. Looking at the list, they can give each column a percentage based on how strongly they feel about each view overall, with the percentages together equaling 100%. The benefits column invariably wins out, which makes clients more likely to let themselves heal from some of their hurtful thoughts.

In reviewing the cost/benefit analysis, make sure you make the point with your clients that the behavior that was hurtful before is not what hurts them now. Rather it is the thoughts they have about it that hurt them now, and those thoughts can be changed.

☑ Activity: Use Quotes for Forgiveness

People generally love quotes, and there are many forgiveness quotes that can help your clients along their journey to healing. Forgiveness quotes are very powerful and can serve as reminders and affirmations.

Displaying quotes on a printed sheet outside your office door, such as in a Plexiglas sign, is a great way to offer short inspirational messages to help your clients grow and heal. Below are some examples of quotes on forgiveness. You might have a sheet of these and others you find on the Internet printed up, and in a group situation you can have everyone pick a favorite quote and explain why. This can be done in individual sessions also, of course. In either scenario, quotes are great springboards for discussion.

A fun way to use quotes for a group activity is to print a number of different ones on a piece of paper, cut the paper into strips (one quote per strip), and put the strips in a hat or bowl. Each participant pulls out a quote and say how it relates to them. This activity can also provide a nice basis for having them make up their own quotes and share them with the group.

Here are some sample quotes on forgiveness:

Forgiveness says you are given another chance to make a new beginning.

—Desmond Tutu

Forgiveness is the fragrance that the violet sheds to the heel that has crushed it.

—Mark Twain

The weak can never forgive. Forgiveness is the attribute of the strong.

—Mahatma Gandhi

Forgiveness is not an occasional act, it is a constant attitude.
—Martin Luther King Jr.

True forgiveness is when you can say, "Thank you for that experience"
—Oprah Winfrey

Resentment is like drinking poison and then hoping it will kill your enemies.
—Nelson Mandela

As I walked out the door toward the gate that would lead to my freedom, I knew if I didn't leave my bitterness and hatred behind, I'd still be in prison.
—Nelson Mandela

Forgiveness is the beginning of a new chapter, not the end of the story.
—Fred Luskin

☑ Activity: Role Play for Forgiveness

There are times when confronting a person whom you feel has wronged you can't happen in real life, but that doesn't mean you can't role-play with your clients to help them work out their resentment. You as the therapist can play the person they are upset with, if you feel your client is emotionally healthy enough to separate feelings about you from those about the other person. Otherwise, you can play the client and the client can play the person who has transgressed.

One of the most poignant scenes that demonstrates the power of re-enactment of a traumatic event occurs in the movie *Ordinary People* (1980), where a troubled teen (played by Timothy Hutton) works out his anger with his therapist (played by Judd Hirsch). The therapist role-plays the part of the teenage brother of his client, who let go of the boat when they were out during a storm, drowning in the boating accident. This enactment becomes the turning point in therapy, allowing Hutton to let go of his anger at his brother for letting go of the boat and drowning, making him feel guilty for letting him drown, and leaving the family broken in the aftermath of his death. This short excerpt from the movie can be played in a group situation, which can easily be found by searching for clips of Ordinary People on YouTube or MovieClips (This can make a real impact and be an excellent catalyst for discussion about the healing power of therapy).

☑ Activity: Developing Healing Rituals

Healing rituals that are so common in religious practices also have a place in healing emotions in the course of psychotherapy. Estelle Frankel (2003) writes of a healing ritual she did with a client whose life did not turn out the way she had envisioned. Her middle-aged client had never married nor had children despite that being her dream. Frankel had this client bring a beautiful vase from home into therapy one session, one that she had cherished. In a ritual of healing, with her therapist looking on, she broke the vase and collected the pieces to make a mosaic out of them. The breaking of the vase symbolized her coming to terms with her shattered vision of how her life would turn out, and this ritual helped her to be ready to move on from that disappointment. This healing ritual could easily be made into a ritual of forgiveness, where clients give up the dream of "a better past." Burning photos and letters, throwing ashes into the ocean, or even burying something symbolic from a relationship turned sour are examples of healing rituals.

Healing rituals do not have to be destructive. Merely lighting a candle is a very calming healing ritual. You might suggest to clients that lighting a small candle and watching it burn down can symbolize the extinction of the hold past hurts have on them as they watch the candle melt away.

A Toolkit of Metaphors for Forgiveness

Band-Aid and ointment. Soothe your wounds with the dressings of forgiveness.

Mosaic piece. Dreams and disappointments that have shattered can be made into something even more beautiful, such as a mosaic. (Mosaic pieces can be bought in packages at a hobby store.)

Candle. Instead of allowing anger to burn inside, allow your resentments to burn on the outside as you watch them melt away.

Beach ball. If you inflate a beach ball and try to push it underwater, it will keep popping back up. If grudges are not dealt with, they will keep popping back up.

A coin. This can serve as a reminder to do a cost/benefit analysis. The coin itself represents the "cost" and both sides of the coin represent the 2 sides of the "cost" and "benefit."

Can you and your client think of any more metaphors? This is a great group activity!

Therapeutic Takeaways

☑ Forgiveness is one of the most misunderstood human acts. Your clients will likely need some education to clear up their misconceptions about forgiveness.

☑ Make sure your clients learns that forgiveness does not mean condoning a behavior, and it does not require the transgressor to be sorry. Rather, forgiveness is a choice and a gift that you give yourself to let yourself—not the other person—"off the hook."

☑ Using Kubler-Ross's five-stages-of-grieving model will help you help your clients through the grieving process.

☑ Using metaphors and visualizations can help your clients forgive.

☑ Bibliotherapy and cinematherapy can be quite useful in helping clients process forgiveness.

☑ A variety of written exercises, such as keeping a "forgiveness log," keeping a journal, making a list of the costs and benefits of forgiveness, or writing a gratitude list, can help your clients heal with forgiveness.

Handouts

The following worksheets will help your clients develop skills for healing themselves with forgiveness. The worksheets are all related to the lessons of this chapter. As a general guideline, handouts and assignments are given to your clients at the end of the session as homework, unless they are used in the session itself to illustrate points. Make sure you leave ample time to go over your expectations regarding the use of the selected handout.

When assignments are given out, it is important to follow up with your clients at the beginning of the next session to review and discuss their homework. Going over the homework is an essential aspect of being a solution-oriented therapist.

Note: All handouts in the book are available for download on my website by following the link below: http://www.belmontwellness.com/ultimate-solution-handouts/

Handout 7.1: Common Myths About Forgiveness

Myth 1: Forgiving means condoning behavior and letting someone off the hook.

Forgiving lets you off the hook—not the other person. It frees you from bitterness and from the past that cannot be altered in the present. When you forgive, you give up the anger and resentment that stops you from healing, but you do not condone the behavior. When you forgive someone, you let go of the expectation that he or she was able to be healthier, and you refuse to be a victim anymore.

Myth 2: Forgiving is mostly a gift you give to others.

Forgiveness is primarily a gift you give to yourself. When you forgive, you accept that a person's unacceptable behavior is due to his or her own limitations, and acknowledge that people cannot give you what they do not have inside. By letting go of the grudge, you let go of your negativity and bitterness—which is like poison to you, not the other person. Letting the negativity go will let you move forward in life without the chains from the past holding you back.

Myth 3: Forgiving means forgetting.

Why would you want to forget something that helped shape you into who you are today? It is much better to learn than to forget, because you will decrease the chances that history will repeat itself. There are times to hold on, and times to let go—and in healing from the past, letting go is not forgetting, but giving up the hold that the memories have over you. When you forget, things are more likely to happen again. When you forgive, but don't go back for more, you can improve your future by keeping in mind lessons from your past.

Myth 4: You can forgive only when you no longer hurt.

There are some things in life that will always hurt, such as the death of a loved one or a traumatic situation where you were completely victimized and had no control. However, that doesn't mean you can't move on and be happy in life despite the hurt. But in order for you to grow from the hurt, you need embrace forgiveness. As actress Lily Tomlin said, "Forgiveness means giving up all hope for a better past."

Myth 5: To be forgiven, the person needs to be sorry.

Those who wait for their transgressors to feel remorse might wait for a lifetime. That gives the transgressor too much power over your ability to heal. Some people are just too mentally crippled to take responsibility for their actions, or have some type of personality disorder, and lack of remorse is one of the hallmarks. They think that their problems are everyone else's fault. When people can't or won't take responsibility for being hurtful, you may need to protect yourself and set good limits, distance yourself, or even completely take them out of your life, depending on the situation. However, you can still exercise forgiveness.

Myth 6: If you forgive, you are being weak and not standing up for your rights.

To the contrary, forgiveness is a sign of strength. Letting going of the control someone has over you requires you to be strong and courageous. Forgiveness allows you to become stronger because of the hurt, not weaker. Through lessons learned and building on the pain to move past the hurt, you will gain strength of character.

As Mahatma Gandhi said, "The weak can never forgive. Forgiveness is the attribute of the strong."

Handout 7.2: Healing Thoughts for Forgiveness

Healing Thoughts for Forgiving Others

1. If you can't forgive, you get stuck in a moment of time. You become a prisoner of your past.
2. You deserve to free yourself from the bitterness that holds you back from a healthier life.
3. Forgiveness frees you from the burden of grudges that hold you back from a more positive life.
4. Forgiveness helps you to let go of old wounds and helps you reclaim your life.
5. Forgiveness is more about you than it is about the other person.
6. Realize that some fences need repair and some fences can't be fixed. Regardless, forgive.
7. Remember that people cannot give you what they don't have in themselves to give.

Healing Thoughts to Forgive Yourself

- It is unfair to look from your vantage point now and expect yourself to know *then* what you know *now*. Forgive yourself for not having the foresight to know what you now know in hindsight.
- Do what you can now to make things right. Let your regrets propel you into positive action, not keep you a prisoner of your past.
- If you need to apologize or make amends, do it now. Admitting fault is a sign of strength, not of weakness.
- It might be too late to change what happened, but it is not too late to change how you cope with what happened, and what you do about it now.
- In reality, most of our stumbles are not failures if we learn from them. They cause us to deepen and become wiser.
- You won't be able to truly forgive others until you can forgive yourself.

Handout 7.3: My Forgiveness Log

A Situation or Person That Needs My Forgiveness	
Negative Emotions	Positive Emotions
Strength of Negative Emotions 1 2 3 4 5 6 7 8 9 10 Low High	Strength of Positive Emotions 1 2 3 4 5 6 7 8 9 10 Low High
Identify Unforgiving Beliefs	Challenge With Forgiving Beliefs
Certainty of Your Beliefs 1 2 3 4 5 6 7 8 9 10 Low High	Certainty of Your Beliefs 1 2 3 4 5 6 7 8 9 10 Low High
Unhealthy Reactions to Holding Grudges	Healthy Reactions to Being Forgiving
Cost/Benefit Analysis of Being Unforgiving	Cost/Benefit Analysis of Forgiveness
My Conclusions and Goals	

Handout 7.4: Journaling for Forgiveness

Think of a person or the action of a person whom you have chosen to work on forgiving. Fill out the following sheet to work through your angry and bitter feelings so that you can reach a point of forgiveness and peace.

Describe what happened.

_____

Describe how and why it hurt.

_____

Describe why it still hurts.

_____

Describe how the hurt has held you back.

_____

Describe your behavioral reaction to the hurt back then.

_____

Describe how your behavior is affected now.

_____

Describe what you have learned from the hurt.

_____

Describe your strategies for healing.

_____

List some behavioral steps you want to take so that you can forgive and move on.

_____

_____

_____

_____

Handout 7.5: The Five Stages of Grieving and Healing
Based on the works of Kubler-Ross (1969)

	Grieving Death	*Grieving From Hurtful Memories*
DENIAL	I will not accept that my loved one is dying. I cannot accept my own mortality.	I will not admit that I am hurt. It's no big deal.
ANGER	I am angry at life's unfairness.	I blame others for hurting me; I can't forgive.
BARGAINING	If only I do something, maybe it won't happen. I might have power to alter what is happening.	Maybe others will "see the light," change their minds, or reconsider, if I can only show them.
DEPRESSION	I was powerless and could not change life's reality. I feel sad and hopeless, and there is nothing I can do.	I can't forgive others for the damage they caused. It's hopeless, and I feel helpless.
ACCEPTANCE	I have prepared for the inevitability of death and have made amends with the important people in my life. I have come to terms with my own mortality and that of my loved ones.	I look forward to growing from the hurt. I will work on acceptance and forgiveness. I will let go of the dreams and expectations that could not come true.

Handout 7.6: Quick Test: What Is Your Forgiveness IQ?

It's not easy to forgive when you feel slighted or wronged, yet we know that the inability to forgive causes us to hold on to bitterness and negativity. For some, forgiving oneself for past actions and choices proves to be the most challenging of all. It is important to keep in mind that forgiveness is a choice and reflects a conscious decision. The first step is to identify the essential elements of forgiveness, which can provide a basis for focusing on the areas that need most attention. The key to interpret your score is on the next page.

For the following 10 questions, rate each item from 1 to 10 to find your "forgiveness IQ."

Strongly Disagree   1   2   3   4   5   6   7   8   9   10   Strongly Agree

_____ I will not forgive people if they are not sorry and admit what they've done.

_____ Those who have wronged or slighted me but take no responsibility for hurting me do not deserve to be forgiven.

_____ I find that my inability to forgive leaves me stuck thinking about what happened in the past.

_____ I can't forgive because I don't want to condone bad behavior.

_____ A difficulty in forgiving makes it hard for me to trust others.

_____ It's hard to forgive, because forgiving means letting people off the hook and makes them no longer accountable.

_____ Forgiveness is something that you just feel, not a trainable skill.

_____ Since there is nothing I can do about things now, I tend to keep things in and don't share my hurt with others.

_____ If I forgive, that means I will be vulnerable again, and I need to protect myself.

_____ I can't forgive myself for past mistakes, choices, and failures.

Total Score: _____

How did you do? The lower the score, the better your forgiveness IQ. The following is a rough guideline for interpreting your score:

15 or lower   You are a forgiveness genius! Congratulations!

16–29   Strong forgiveness competency. You have given yourself the gift of forgiveness and stay positive.

30–49   Moderate forgiveness competency. You have some work to do on becoming less negative and stuck in past resentments.

50–69   Moderate forgiveness impairment. A difficulty with forgiveness has limited your ability to stay positive and live fully in the present.

70–84   Severe forgiveness impairment. Consider seeking professional help to give yourself the gift of forgiveness.

85–100   DANGER ZONE! A lack of forgiveness impairs your mental health. Consider seeking psychological help.

Handout 7.7: Weekly Forgiveness Log

Date(s): _____

1. What I have trouble forgiving:

_____

2. Emotional response to my difficulty forgiving:

_____

3. Degree of my negative reaction:

    LOW 1 2 3 4 5 6 7 8 9 10 HIGH

4. Unhealthy thoughts:

_____

    Certainty of beliefs: LOW 1 2 3 4 5 6 7 8 9 10 HIGH

5. Healthy thoughts:

_____

    Certainty of beliefs: LOW 1 2 3 4 5 6 7 8 9 10 HIGH

6. Unhealthy reactions to being unforgiving:

_____

7. Healthy reactions to forgiveness   :

_____

8. Metaphors and visualizations I use to forgive:

_____

9. Costs and benefits of my healthy and unhealthy thinking:

_____

10. Goal for working on my forgiveness and improving my coping skills:

_____

Recommended Resources

Self-help Books

The Four Things That Matter Most: A Book About Living
    Ira Byock
The Choosing to Forgive Workbook: Discove Contentment and Peace
    by Letting Go of Harmful Anger
    Les Carter and Frank Minirth
On Death and Dying
    Elisabeth Kubler-Ross
Life Lessons: Two Experts on Death & Dying Teach Us About the Mysteries of Life & Living
    Elisabeth Kubler-Ross and David Kessler
Forgive for Good: A Proven Prescription for Health and Happiness
    Fred Luskin

Links

Cognitive Behaviour Therapy Self-Help Resources
    http://www.getselfhelp.co.uk/freedownloads2.htm
Forgive for Good
(Fred Luskin's site)
    http://learningtoforgive.com
The Forgiveness Project
    http://theforgivenessproject.com
Kim's Counseling Corner
"Therapeutic & Self-Help Worksheets"
    http://www.kimscounselingcorner.com/resources/therapy-and-self
    -help-worksheets/
Psychology Tools
("Forgiveness" self-help worksheets and handouts)
    http://www.psychologytools.org/forgiveness.html

CHAPTER EIGHT

The Low Self-Esteem Solution
Busting Core Irrational Beliefs

Very few of us go through life without some degree of self-doubt and self-critiquing, but often our clients—who come to us with symptoms of depression, anxiety, or substance abuse—are plagued by persistent underlying negative self-evaluations.

Core irrational beliefs typically arise from all-consuming negative self-judgments such as "I'm not good enough," "I am flawed," or "I'm a loser." These negative core beliefs serve as filters that cloud our clients' world and how they see themselves in relation to it. With these negative self-evaluations, deep feelings of shame and guilt add insult to injury.

This negative self-preoccupation leads to extreme self-consciousness in social situations that can affect interpersonal relationships, leading to anything from social isolation and shyness to extreme neediness and dependence.

Low self-esteem is analogous to having a compromised immune system or low resistance to colds or the flu. It provides a breeding ground for all types of secondary problems, such as disturbances in mood and anxiety, as well as other clinical manifestations, such as substance abuse, eating disorders, and body dysmorphia.

In clients with mood and anxiety disorders, low self-esteem is often lurking right below the surface, characterized by distorted self-perceptions and negative thoughts. From a faulty self-image to a rigid, irrational, and self-absorbed self-view in relation to the world, low self-esteem leads to a lack of trust in others reflecting one's own insecurity. Consequently, people with low self-esteem have trouble communicating well with others, tend to be non-assertive and keep too much inside, fearing rejection and criticism. This insecurity and fear of rejection leads to a vicious cycle in which our clients are consumed with self-doubt, and tend to not express their fears and thoughts so that they never reach the light of day and objective self-evaluation. Instead, the fears and perceptions tend to escalate in magnitude, leading our clients further down the path of isolation, anxiety, and self-flagellation, rendering their negative cognitive self-distortions highly resistant to logic and change.

In the case of clients with low self-esteem, no behavioral tools and experiential activities can offer much hope for healing without a strong foundation of safety and positive regard. With this foundation in mind, a solution-oriented therapist needs to go a bit more patiently in treatment with a client with low self-esteem than with a client with a higher sense of self-esteem intact, because the chance of misinterpretations and sensitivity to rejection is so high. I have often been struck by how many ways my clients with low self-esteem interpret my comments in a self-downing way, finding evidence to support their own negative self-view. The types of cognitive distortions that fill their own heads are played out in the therapy session, yet due to their frequent non-assertiveness, they often keep these distortions to themselves, causing a great deal of treatment resistance. I have gotten around this stalemate by becoming very aware of some of my client's nonverbal expressions, noting changes in affect, and I ask them about their reactions to things said in the session, inviting them to give me feedback. I offer many openings to express what's bothering them, if anything, about our discussion, and only with direct questioning do I find out what they are reacting to is frequently their own internal dialogue. For example, on quite a few occasions, clients have viewed my offer to space out appointments not as a "reward" for their progress but as a sign of rejection and validation of their fear that they are not "good" clients.

Once the therapeutic relationship is established with plenty of therapeutic TLC and unconditional, nonjudgmental support, clients with low self-esteem can make the best use out of the strategies provided. With this emotionally nurturing foundation, low self-esteem is treatable with the tools of today's Cognitive Behavior Therapy (CBT) strategies as well as acceptance techniques that emphasize being non-judgmental and mindful. With interventions, clients can learn to be more self-accepting, begin to think more rationally about themselves, and develop more self-compassion. In a sense, the therapist becomes a teacher of a new emotional language, helping clients to interpret the world in a new way that is not based on shame.

Thus, if clients are to like themselves more, they initially need to learn that new emotional language. They might have learned shame-based thinking from parents and other family members, teachers, peers at school, or other influential people in their lives. They might have arrived at faulty conclusions about themselves from those who did not know any better, whether resulting from their own misperceptions or in reaction to the misperceptions of others. Therapists have the unique opportunity to enlighten their clients to the fact that this first shame-based language was actually more like Pig Latin than a bona fide language.

Lauren was a 72-year-old woman who lived with her husband, her divorced 38-year-old daughter, and her 10-year-old grandchild. She came to counseling for support, as she felt as if no one at home except her grandchild respected her. She claimed that her husband hollered at her frequently, which triggered distinct memories of her long deceased father's loud voice. She felt that since her father, husband, and daughter kept on finding fault with her, maybe she really was not a good person. She also wondered if she was just too old to change. Her self-esteem was very low, and any compliments I gave her were a source of embarrassment and surprise. She wasn't used to anyone saying anything positive about her, and she wasn't in the habit of saying positive things to herself. She asked me how her father, husband, and daughter could all be so wrong, and since they all concurred with each other, she feared that they were right about her. Her self-esteem was so low that at one session when I told her that we could meet in two weeks instead of one, since things seemed to be going much better, she looked at me with a saddened expression and said, "I guess I'm not a very good patient, am I?" Through the filter of her distorted self-view, she immediately decided that I was just going to give myself a break for the week by avoiding her.

Another client, Jill, was a 44-year-old married mother of three. She claimed that, having grown up in a very dogmatic and fervently religious household, she felt as if *sin* was her middle name. She was constantly critiqued for being "selfish," "sinful," and "lazy." In considering divorce from her husband after years in an unhappy marriage, her family told her she would be sinning against God, and she lived with guilt and bad feelings about herself. In looking for approval from her family, she gave up what she saw was her only shot at a happy life. She remained in an unhappy marriage with a husband who was also constantly putting her down, and she found herself having panic attacks and bouts of depression. Worrying about what her parents and other people would think if she left her husband, and having found out that no matter how much she stood up to her husband he would be rude and verbally abusive to her, she ended up overeating and becoming more and more depressed because she felt as if there was no way out.

These two examples describe clients who learned a faulty, shame-based first language from their families of origin. The first tip in this following treatment tips section offers some guidance for clinicians on how to see themselves as emotional translators for their clients. Learning a new emotional language is essential to revamping negative self-talk that undermines self-esteem and growth.

Treatment Tips

☑ Mini-Lesson: The Therapist as Translator
and Language Teacher

When clients come to therapy with impaired self-esteem, the therapist assumes the role of an emotional translator and teacher, teaching clients a new, healthier emotional language. Their first shame-based language taught them that other people could make or break their self-esteem, and that evaluative and negative judgments by others were correct and could determine their self-worth. When a client needs encouragement and reassurance to change ingrained shame-based thinking, I use the analogy of how people who have relocated to the United States from other countries often retain their accents—despite living in the U.S. for decades—and keep their first language as their "default." Even though some people have only a trace of a different accent after being assimilated into U.S. culture, they claim to still think and/or dream in their native language.

It is liberating for clients to learn that they no longer have to be defined by that erroneous language. If clients become impatient with their progress, I reassure them that it is as if they had learned Pig Latin for decades before deciding to get therapy, and that it will take some time to translate ideas into a healthier language. With this analogy, clients feel a sense of freedom, open themselves up to a world of new possibilities, and become kinder and more patient with themselves. Reassure your clients that no matter how difficult it is for them to learn a new language, if they use a mix of practice, hope, and trust, it is only a matter of time before they will become fluent!

☑ Mini-Lesson: Helping Clients Identify Faulty Equations

For clients who suffer with low self-esteem—who interpret things in extremely skewed, negative ways—I use the analogy of a math equation, suggesting that the way they are adding things up in their heads is faulty. Instead of 1 plus 1 equals 2, or even 11 (in their way of thinking), their equation is more like 1 plus 1 equals 457 regarding how they jump to conclusions about events in their lives.

Clients typically enjoy this analogy and find humor in the absurdity of their errors, and this becomes a running joke. For example, if the logic is a bit more grounded, I bring the numbers down to 1 plus 1 equals 127. When the logic is way out of whack, the numbers sometimes go into the thousands.

Eventually, when clients recognize their own distorted thinking, they begin to use this analogy themselves and learn to laugh at their faulty self-appraisals. This is an especially good thing, since one of the problems with low self-esteem is that people take themselves way too seriously, and using the new language or math equations analogy provides a great metaphorical tool to help them lighten up and thus to improve their self-esteem.

☑ Demonstration: Your Self-Worth Remains

Having an emotionally safe and nonjudgmental relationship with your clients will help them to be less judgmental of themselves. Being kind and compassionate as a therapist encourages your clients to be compassionate toward themselves. Creating an atmosphere of acceptance is especially important, as clients with low self-esteem often enter therapy with many insecurities and the fear that they will not be accepted or— even worse—that they will be actively rejected. They don't want to be thought of as a "bad" client. Within the atmosphere of what Carl Rogers called "unconditional positive regard (1989)," cognitive restructuring, mindfulness activities, visualizations, and demonstrations will help your clients cultivate loving-kindness toward themselves.

One short and powerful demonstration that I use with clients individually and in groups demonstrates this non-judgmental acceptance. No matter what they have gone through, or how bad they feel about themselves, their self-worth remains. Using the example of a large dollar bill ask your clients to do whatever they want with it, as long as they don't destroy it or render it unusable since you need it for food shopping later in the day! Clients fold it, step on it, crumble it, and so forth, and then when it comes back to you, flatten it so that it looks again like the bill you started with. Make the point that some bills are new and crispy, while some are old and worn. In a group situation, after everyone has taken a turn, or your individual client has taken as many turns as he or she likes, unfold the bill and ask how much it is now worth. The idea is that regardless of how crumpled or worn the bill is, it still retains its worth.

The analogy from this demonstration is very powerful, illustrating that despite how worn and crumpled we feel—and regardless of what has happened to us—our self-worth is not altered, and we are still just as valuable. This is a very powerful exercise for children and adults alike, and they are often reminded of its message each time they handle money.

☑ Activity: Mirror, Mirror on the Wall

This exercise is designed to help clients stop judging themselves by unrealistic standards and instead focus on more positive ones by using others they admire as a yardstick of how kindly they can view themselves.

Begin by asking your clients to look in the mirror and write down what they see. Usually clients with low self-esteem choose their unfavorable physical aspects. Write down what your clients report, and then ask your clients to look away from the mirror to finish the list with attributes about themselves. Most often, this list continues to be negative. Some examples I have heard are, "I have a big nose," I have too many wrinkles," and "I hate my hair."

Then ask your clients who they most admire and have them write down the same number of characteristics for that person as they mentioned for themselves. This list is typically more focused on the inner qualities of being a kind and good person rather than on outer qualities or human imperfections. For instance, a client might say, "She is kind, warm, and loving."

Compare the two lists, and offer the suggestion that perhaps they needs to regard their own inner qualities like they do those of others. Point out to clients that they often view others more kindly and gently, while being harder on themselves by focusing too heavily on their exaggerated dislike of their physical characteristics.

This is a great springboard for the Cognitive Behavior Therapy (CBT) technique popularized by David Burns: the Double Standard Technique.

☑ Demonstration: The Double Standard Technique

In the Double Standard Technique, clients are first urged to recognize that they have a double standard for themselves and the rest of the world. They may harshly condemn themselves for things regarding which they would be compassionate toward others. For example, a group participant who feels unlikable and unpopular might equate people not being attracted to her as proof that she is inferior and a failure. However, if you asked this client to describe others she knows who also have few friends and are unpopular, the description would be much kinder and compassionate, such as that this person is *shy* instead of being a *loser*.

Diane was a 41-year-old client who was very hard on herself for her promiscuous past before she got married. Twenty years later, she still felt it defined her as a "whore," and it interfered with her relationship with her husband and clouded her feelings about herself.

I asked Diane to think of a female in her life whom she admired; she chose her boss. I questioned her as to whether, if she knew that her boss had a similar promiscuous past, would she think of her as a whore? She appeared to be taken aback and claimed it would not change her opinion of her boss at all. She thought her boss was awesome, and if that was in her past then Diane would be even more impressed that she became the person she was today after having made so many poor choices. I then asked my client why she could not draw the same conclusion about herself.

To demonstrate this Double Standard Technique in a role-play within a group setting, David Burns combines it with another technique called the "Externalization of Voices." In this technique, the leader or someone in the group acts like a monstrously absurd figure who exaggerates the negative self-talk of the person with the double standard. Examples include "You are the biggest loser in the world," while the subject will defend himself or herself with more positive answers, just as he or she would defend anyone else. Having the exaggerated negative thoughts played out by the external voice (played by the group leader or another group member) will help all group members see how illogical this double standard is for people with low self-esteem. If you feel that a client's self-esteem is too fragile to allow them to hear these exaggerations without becoming upset, you can have the client play the monstrous character while you play the positive, more rational voice of the client defending against the absurd accusations.

Here is an example of how such a dialogue might play out:

THERAPIST AS CLIENT: I make a lot of mistakes at work sometimes, and I am afraid they think I am stupid.
CLIENT PLAYING THE MONSTROUSLY ABSURD VOICE: "You are dumber than a doorknob—of course they think you are the dumbest worker they ever had. They'll probably fire you tomorrow when you come in."

THERAPIST AS CLIENT: "I am not *that* stupid—that's silly. A lot of my coworkers make mistakes too."

The Double Standard Technique and the Externalization of Voices techniques demonstrate how techniques can be combined techniques to make them more powerful than each alone. You can also do this activity with a private client, although demonstration is ideal and has a more powerful impact in a group. References for David Burns' powerful combination of these two techniques are included in the resources section at the end of this chapter.

☑ Demonstration: Self-Esteem (Torn Apart)

In this demonstration—which is very effective for both individual clients and groups—use a piece of paper as a visual for self-worth and self-esteem. Show a full piece of paper to your clients to illustrate the fact that we begin life with the capacity for a complete sense of self-esteem. But somehow along the way, some of us develop low self-esteem and get the idea that we are somehow "not good," "wrong," "selfish," "unlikable," "lazy," "fat," and "unworthy." As you say each of those words, take off a little piece of the paper to demonstrate little pieces of self-esteem being torn apart from the "whole" sense of self. You might then say something like, "Some of us get those messages from parents or other family members who were treated that way themselves and didn't know any better. Some of us got more subtle messages that we weren't good enough from our families of origins—perhaps from well-meaning parents who just were trying their best to motivate us to be the best we could be, leaving us to feel we were not good enough. Others of us got the idea we were not good enough because we were made fun of and even bullied in school. Thus, bombarded with so many unhealthy and invalidating messages, we end up walking around in life as just a shred of what we could have been and could be." Continue to tear off another piece of paper as you give each example, until by the end only a remnant of paper remains. "Some people walk around through life like this ragged, small piece of paper."

I often use this demonstration with my individual clients with low self-esteem. It is very powerful to see a visual representation of a torn sense of self. Another variation is to keep the paper intact and just crease it.

To further the exercise, especially when the paper is just creased and not torn, show your clients that the paper can be flattened and remains whole despite the creases. Or with tape, you can put a shredded paper back together (you can actually do this during group sessions). While there may be imperfections, every piece can be saved.

Ask your clients questions to help them process this activity, such as, "What fraction of a whole piece are you dealing with today? How much can you put back together?" Each person can then take pieces off their own sheet of paper and hold up what's left. Those with low self-esteem have a smaller piece remaining than those with a strong sense of self.

☑ Demonstration: Self-Esteem is Like an Egg

Sometimes for a visual impact, especially in a group, I bring in an egg to symbolize that we all are fragile and need to handle ourselves with care. We don't want to get too hard-boiled, but we need to protect ourselves (as with an eggshell) from feeling too vulnerable, like a raw egg that cannot withstand much abuse. I also use the egg in describing how we need to handle our relationships with care (described in Chapter 6), but in the case of low self-esteem, we need to take care of ourselves first. Many people with low self-esteem are more concerned about handling others with care but aren't so nice to themselves in terms of their self-talk and beliefs about themselves. Having clients take turns holding the egg and saying one kind thing about themselves can be an effective way of unlocking positive self-talk and self-compassion.

☑ Mindfulness Solutions: Helping Your Clients Boost Their Self-Esteem

The mindfulness strategies of the third-wave approaches are ideal for building self-esteem, since they are geared toward self-compassion and self-acceptance. In addition, so much of our clients' low self-esteem originates from past choices, the past messages they received, and the regrets they feel based on their past actions. The mindfulness approach focuses only on the present, helping clients to be aware of present sensations with a nonjudgmental stance. The following are a few examples of the mindfulness approach as it is applied to the treatment of low self-esteem.

Marsha Linehan's Dialectical Behavior Therapy (DBT) model focuses on four main areas, and one of them is *radical acceptance*. This is a practice in which there is radical (or total) acceptance of what is, rather than fighting against it. This acceptance is also done with complete suspension of the judgment that whatever we knew as terrible, awful, and so forth just *is*. Practicing radical acceptance is consciously observing with a "Teflon mind" to which thoughts don't stick—they just come and go. Instruct your clients to observe their judgments and thoughts, but not get too attached to them. Linehan suggests that this mindful practice be done through daily activities, not necessarily in a meditative position. Washing the dishes, cleaning the bathroom, and taking a walk are all opportunities to develop radical acceptance though non-judgmental mindfulness. The key is to do one thing at a time, in the present moment, with full awareness of sensations like sounds, smells, sights, and so forth.

But does this relate to self-esteem? A lot! Since self-esteem is low due to negative self-evaluations, this concept does away with the mind's judgmental stance so that the negative self-evaluations are just observed in a detached way. In other chapters in this book, we learned that the art of mindfully describing and observing is accomplished by focusing on observable facts, such as "His lips are pursed and his brow is furrowed," rather than judgments, such as "He is furious!" The first is an observation, the latter an interpretation that has various shades of truth and is subject to debate. Saying that "the sky has many clouds" is a nonjudgmental description; saying that "the weather is lousy" is a judgment. As it relates to a negative thought, a mindful and accepting stance would be "I am having the thought that I am a failure" rather than "I am a failure." This distinction is very important, because one interpretation is an imparted observation, while the other is a judgment.

By performing mindfulness practices such as these, clients will get in the habit of being present focused and feeling sensations with all their senses rather than getting wrapped up in their own internal mental events.

☑ ACT Technique: Hand Exercise

ACT founder Steven Hayes's metaphoric exercise for mindfulness is a simple one to use with your clients. Have your clients put their hands in front of their eyes, blocking what is around them. Instruct them to lower their hands so they can see around them through their fingers. Allowing just a little space to look through, their fingers represent our negative misperceptions that block our vision and interfere with our ability to be clearly mindful of the present. Literally and figuratively, fingers before our eyes obscure our ability to be present focused, and the fingers represent the thoughts and judgments that get in the way. This demonstration can be very powerful with your clients when discussing low self-esteem. Negative self-talk prevents us from experiencing the moment as it is, it clouds our judgment, and it obscures our self-view, symbolized by fingers before our eyes.

☑ ACT Technique: The Quicksand Metaphor

This metaphor, also created by Steven Hayes, can be used in the treatment of many different problems, including low self-esteem.

Using the image of quicksand, Hayes states that the immediate impulse most people have is to struggle and fight to get out. However, by fighting the quicksand, you just sink in deeper, and the more you struggle, the deeper you go. The only way to resist sinking deeper in the quicksand is to surrender to it—to stop fighting it and lay outstretched on top of it, spreading your weight over the surface so you won't sink. Likewise, the less you accept yourself, the more you judge, and the farther you sink into the figurative quicksand. By accepting your struggles instead of fighting to change what can't be changed, you actually end up less stuck and won't sink in deeper.

☑ DBT Technique: Self-Soothing Practice

In DBT, there is an emphasis on developing self-soothing skills that relax both the hurt and the self-destructive feelings that accompany low self-esteem (Linehan, 1993). Helping your clients create a list of soothing behaviors—such as lighting candles, taking a bubble bath, or being more mindful of the present moment through the use of their five senses—

encourages them to heal through present awareness instead of judgmental perseveration.

Help them develop a self-soothing kit to remind them of how to take care of themselves during stressful times. Whether this kit is a tangible one or a virtual one on the computer, your clients will be reminded that they deserve to take care of themselves.

☑ DBT Technique: Using Acronyms to Replace Old Skills

DBT is rich in acronyms that stand for various skills for clients to practice. The IMPROVE acronym, for instance, helps structure your clients' pursuit of being more mindful, accepting, and focused on the present.

> *Imagine:* Imagine a peaceful scene and listen to relaxing and soothing music while your harmful self-talk and emotions drain out of your mind like water out of a pipe.
>
> *Meaning:* Discover the meaning in your adversities—everything can help you grow if you let it!
>
> *Prayer:* Ask for help from a higher spiritual power, or even others—there is hope!
>
> *Relaxation:* Take a slow, deep breath. Practicing slow breathing will calm you down and increase your oxygen intake.
>
> *Mindfulness:* Take a nonjudgmental focus on the present. Accept life as it is, and accept yourself too.
>
> *Vacation:* Take time for yourself by enjoying a mini-break, even if it's only for a couple of minutes.
>
> *Encouragement:* Be your own cheerleader by saying nice things to yourself.

☑ ACT Technique: Cognitive Defusion

Cognitive defusion is an acceptance technique from Steven Hayes, who uses this term to mean distancing your negative thoughts from your mind. He reasons that negative self-evaluations are so often "fused" in our clients' minds that only by performing cognitive defusion practices can they separate their minds from their negative self-talk.

The approach of Acceptance and Commitment Therapy (ACT) is full of metaphors and visualizations. One of Hayes's best-known visualizations of cognitive defusion is "leaves on a stream." In this visualization, clients are asked to imagine themselves by a stream, putting their negative thoughts about themselves on separate leaves and watching them float away and eventually disappear down the stream. The key to cognitive defusion is to distance yourself from your thoughts by looking *at* them, not *from* them.

This leaves-on-a-stream image has been very effective in treating resistant clients who have experienced only limited success with CBT techniques, especially those who possess deeply ingrained low self-esteem from mentally or physically abusive childhoods. This same type of exercise can be used with other images, such as watching clouds in the sky, each of which contains your clients' negative self-labels. By watching them from afar, clients release these labels and stop keeping them inside their heads.

Hayes also uses the metaphor of standing on a bridge watching as trains go under it. He has his readers imagine that each of their disturbing thoughts are on a separate train car by watching them go by will help readers look *at* their disturbing thoughts, not *from* them.

☑ CBT Technique: Coping Cards

Encourage your clients to use coping cards to remind them of their worth. Affirmations written on the cards may include things like "I am good enough" and "I am a beautiful human being."

You can suggest to your clients that they use their affirmation coping cards as the basis for a ritual every morning in which they look into the mirror and repeat their affirmations. I had one client who claimed that this ritual actually changed her life. Each morning before work she looked in the mirror and engaged in this ritual of self-love. One of her affirmations was that she deserved to be happy, and she was going to choose to be happy—she was worthy. She repeated this every morning, and she was amazed at how soothing this ritual was and how it helped her to solidify her self-esteem.

"Coping Card Ideas" (Handout 8.2) offers various examples of coping cards to show your client. This will give your clients ideas for making up their own.

☑ CBT Technique: The Triple-Column Technique

All CBT researchers and authors use some type of log for recording automatic thoughts and replacing them with more adaptive thoughts. There are endless variations of CBT logs and journals for clients to use to pinpoint their unhealthy thoughts and replace them with healthier ones. They are commonly referred to as thought records, daily mood logs, thought journals, thought logs, dysfunctional thought records, or thoughts/feelings awareness logs, to name a few.

A CBT thought log by David Burns (1999) is a popular example. It contains the elements of most of the widely used CBT thought record formats and is one of the four components of Burns' widely used Daily Mood Log, in which irrational thoughts about oneself are replaced by more rational thoughts.

Here is a description of the three columns used in the triple-column technique:

Column 1. Write an automatic negative thought, rating the degree of your certainty of the belief from 0 to 100.
Column 2. Identify the type of cognitive error from a checklist of cognitive distortions.
Column 3. Respond to the distortion with a more rational thought, rating the degree of your certainty of the belief from 0 to 100.

Here is an example of the triple-column technique in action:

Negative Thought	Type of Cognitive Distortion	Rational Response
I keep goofing up	*All-or-nothing thinking,*	*I do many things right*
70% certainty	*overgeneralization*	*80% certainty*

Since the log uses cognitive distortions, I have listed below, for your convenience, many of the cognitive distortions that characterize illogical thoughts.

- All-or-nothing thinking
- Comparing

- Jumping to conclusions
- Blaming
- "Should" statements
- Overgeneralization
- Mental filter
- Mind reading
- Selective or emotional reasoning
- Fortune telling
- Magnification or minimization
- Emotional reasoning
- Personalization

In the handouts section, I have also offered many other types of thought logs, such as "My Thoughts/Feelings/Behavior Log" (Handout 8.4), a variation based on the triple-column technique. "My Self-Esteem Log" (Handout 8.5) is yet another variation of a thought log for your therapeutic toolbox.

☑ CBT Technique: Eradicate the ANTs

Psychologist Daniel Amen (1998) uses the term ANTs to refer to CBT's concept of *automatic negative thoughts*. These ANTs permeate our perceptions so automatically that we are often not even aware of them. The goal of therapy is to uncover core automatic thoughts and dispute them.

An example of an ANT is when my client said, "I am just a klutz." She was told this as a child, her husband agreed, and she treated this like fact. She figured that all of them could not be wrong! I observed that although she tripped occasionally and spilled water, it hardly defined her as a "klutz." I also told her that I do the same at times, and never thought of myself as a "klutz." I asked if she thought I was one, now that she knew I also spilled water and tripped, and she claimed that of course she did not see me like that.

"Recognizing Your ANTs (Automatic Negative Thoughts)" (Handout 8.3) can help your client create a new improved self-view by replacing their negative thoughts with more positive ones. You can help them tackle their ANTs by having them write down—and then respond to—

these distorted put-downs with more self-compassionate thoughts. They can then read them in the session and possibly even record them on their cell phones to play back whenever they need reinforcement.

☑ Activity: Jar of Joy

Create a "Jar of Joy" that includes affirmations, positive quotes, and positive ideas written on strips of paper. Have your clients select one from the jar during each session and then explain why they think what they read is true and how it applies to them. Examples of affirmations to include in the jar are "I am a person who tries my best and I am proud of that," "I am a good person," and "I am proud of how far I have come and what I have learned."

☑ CBT Technique: Vertical or Downward Arrow Technique

The vertical or downward arrow technique is a very popular CBT technique popularized by Robert Leahy, David Burns, and Judith Beck. It is designed to uncover core beliefs that lead to low self-esteem. It has been mentioned in a couple of other chapters but is worth repeating here, as this method is so effective in getting to the core of your client's low self-esteem.

Following is an actual example of how the downward arrow technique was used with a client who was trying to decide whether or not to attend her college reunion.

CLIENT: Going to my college reunion will make me feel embarrassed.

↓THERAPIST: Why would it bother you? What would it mean if that really happened?

CLIENT: They would think I am fat and unattractive.

↓THERAPIST: Why would it bother you? What would it mean if that really happened?

CLIENT: They would feel sorry for me that my life turned out so poorly.

↓THERAPIST: Why would it bother you? What would it mean if that really happened?

CLIENT: They would know that I never amounted to much. I just can't go there.

↓THERAPIST: Why would it bother you? What would it mean if that really happened?

CLIENT: It would remind me that I failed in my life.

Within a matter of minutes, my client and I were able to have a very meaningful discussion concerning her feelings of being a failure. Despite an advanced degree and a prestigious university appointment, she regarded herself as a failure, partly because she felt unattractive and had never married.

☑ CBT Technique: The Acceptance Paradox

Another technique mentioned in other chapters bears repeating briefly, as this technique is such an important tool for dealing with clients with low self-worth. David Burns has made the acceptance paradox a common CBT technique for helping clients to reduce their harsh self-judgment. In this paradoxical technique, Burns encourages clients to agree with their negative thought, but not give it so much power.

For example, if clients feel they made a terrible mistake, they need to agree with the negative thought and just respond with self-talk that says, "Okay, so I made a mistake, but it doesn't mean that I'm a bad person. It means I am human, and I can learn from it." This can be very liberating for clients who blame themselves and see themselves through the lens of shame-based thinking. Basically, it allows clients to accept that some of the imperfections are true, but that we are all works in progress: "So what? What else is new? Excuse me for not knowing this when I was five!"

☑ CBT Technique: Recording Thoughts

Judith Beck (2011) suggests that in addition to having your clients record their thoughts on paper—and then challenge them in a CBT thought log—you can have them record some irrational thoughts and then answer them more rationally on a recorder or smartphone. Using this technique, these thoughts and responses can be played back often throughout the week to help clients stay on track.

Here is one example:

Recording: I'm stupid.
Followed by: I sometimes do things without thinking, but that doesn't mean I am a stupid person. Rather, I am human.

Imagine an old-fashioned tape recorder in your head, with a message that keeps repeating, "I'm worthless," and "I'm a loser." While these negative self-evaluations are so automatic that clients often don't realize that they are nurturing them, they can only break free from them when they stop the recording and replace it with a healthier version.

A Toolkit of Metaphors for Treating Low Self-Esteem

Alphabet flash cards. Clients can remember that they are learning a new language—away from their shame-based first language.

Math flash card: Thought distortions are like saying 1 plus 1 equals 437—it just doesn't add up!

Dollar bill: No matter how many times you crush or wrinkle a bill, it still has the same self-worth. Likewise, your self-worth never inherently changes.

Picture of an arrow. Printing or drawing a picture of an arrow on a notecard can remind your client of the downward arrow technique, with which they can get to the bottom of their core irrational beliefs that erode their self-esteem.

Magnifying glass. This reminds clients to look behind their negative self-evaluations and look closer at their distorted thoughts, replacing them with healthier alternatives. In other words, they can be a *thought detective.*

Therapeutic Takeaways

☑ Clients with a first emotional language of shame-based thinking can learn a new emotionally based language with the therapist as translator and educator.

☑ There are many effective demonstrations to do with individual and group clients to emphasize that our self-worth remains the same, no matter what we do or what happens to us.

☑ Visualizations, metaphors, demonstrations, and activities are all psychoeducational methods for unlocking healthy self-esteem.

☑ Acceptance and mindfulness practices based on third-wave approaches help clients accept themselves without judgment.

☑ Cognitive defusion exercises help clients distance themselves from their unhealthy thoughts by looking *at* their negative self-evaluations rather than *from* them.

☑ CBT offers various types of thought logs and techniques, such as identifying your ANTs, the triple-column technique, and the downward arrow approach, to help clients get to the core of their irrational beliefs.

Handouts

The following worksheets will help your clients build their self-esteem. These worksheets are all related to the lessons of this chapter. As a general guideline, handouts and assignments are given to clients at the end of the session as homework, unless they are used in the session itself to illustrate points. Make sure you leave ample time to go over your expectations regarding the use of the selected handouts.

When assignments are given out, it is important to follow up with your clients at the beginning of the next session by reviewing and discussing their homework with them. Going over the homework is an essential aspect of being a solution-oriented therapist.

Note: All handouts in the book are available for download on my website by following the link below: http://www.belmontwellness.com/ultimate-solution-handouts/

Handout 8.1: Common Myths About Self-Esteem

Myth 1: Too much self-esteem is not good; it makes one appear too self-centered and cocky.

There is no such thing as too much healthy self-esteem. Self-esteem is feeling good about and liking yourself regardless of how flawed and imperfect you may be. It doesn't mean you think you are perfect and better than others, but rather that you value yourself.

Just as flight attendants caution that you must put on your own mask before helping small children in an emergency, you need to take care of yourself before you can take care of others. The more you like yourself, the more you can give to others—*there is just more positive stuff to give!* Cockiness is more about thinking you are better than someone else and is actually a sign of insecurity, not self-esteem.

Myth 2: Self-esteem fluctuates with mood.

True self-esteem is a constant, whether you are in a bad mood or a good mood. Even if you are in a bad mood, your evaluation of yourself doesn't need to change. Feelings of self-esteem are constant, although they can increase over time with a concerted effort to relinquish some of the barriers that interfere with self-esteem.

Myth 3: The more you praise a child, the more self-esteem he or she will have.

This is true only up to a point, and it depends on the type of praise. For example, if someone is told she is really smart because she earned an A, how will she feel when she gets a C?

Self-esteem cannot be contingent upon evaluations based solely on success, as life ensures that each of us will experience significant failure as well. Our intelligence, goodness, or attractiveness should not depend on the evaluations and praise of others. Conversely, if a child is not praised in a healthy manner and is constantly put down, his or her baseline self-esteem will surely suffer. Unconditional acceptance is the best way to ensure healthy self-esteem.

Myth 4: Self-esteem is something you either have or don't have.

In general, the more self-esteem we possess, the healthier we feel and the happier we are. Self-esteem can certainly increase as we dispel old myths about ourselves that we might have adopted from judgmental parents or classmates. And it decreases as we are shunned or face disapproval from people in our lives, such as our boss or our spouse.

Myth 5: Self-esteem is correlated with wealth, looks and brains.

Although prettier, smarter, and wealthier people appear to have enviable lives, these things are not necessarily correlated with self-esteem. None of these factors will ensure high self-esteem, although they may help slightly. What is important is having unconditional self-regard and a positive support system that allows you to feel loved and capable of loving.

Handout 8.2: Coping Card Ideas

One-sided cards: Examples

I am worthy and lovable.
I am a good person and trying the best I can.
Even if I am anxious and get panicky, it is not dangerous.
The most important person to approve of me is me!
Even if I make a mistake, it does not mean I am a failure—it means I am human.
I deserve a happy life.

Two-sided cards

I have too many issues.	These experiences will help me be a deeper and more compassionate person.
I am too fat.	I am working on my diet and exercise, and I am proud of the steps I am taking.
I am unlikable.	Not everyone will like me; it is most important that I like myself.
I can't stand to be criticized.	The opinions of others do not define my self-worth.
I'll never be comfortable presenting at meetings.	I will keep practicing and rehearsing and remain committed to the subject I know best.
He makes me so mad.	I am in charge at how mad I get—he does not need to have so much control over me.
I can't stand it!	I can stand it—I just don't like it.

Handout 8.3: Recognizing Your ANTs
(Automatic Negative Thoughts)

Remember: You CAN eradicate the ANTs! This concept is based on the work of psychiatrist Daniel Amen, author of "Change Your Brain, Change Your Life."

Automatic Negative Thought (ANT)	Type of ANT Distortion

13 Types of ANT Distortions That Lead to Low Self-Esteem

1. *Catastrophizing.* You label things as horrible and awful instead of unfortunate and disappointing: *"This is HORRIBLE!"*
2. *Fortune telling.* You think you can predict the future: *"I'll never find anyone who will be interested in me. I'll be alone the rest of my life."*
3. *Black-and-white thinking.* You make all-or-nothing assumptions: *"No men are trustworthy."*
4. *Personalization.* You blame yourself for things that are out of your control: *"I am to blame for my child's issues."*
5. *Jumping to conclusions.* You make assumptions and regard them as fact: *"He told me that he couldn't come to the party because he just doesn't like me."*
6. *Labeling.* You label yourself and others instead of being specific: *Instead of saying, "I made a mistake," you label yourself a "failure" or a "loser."*
7. *Magnification.* You make mountains out of molehills: *"This is the worst day of my life!"*
8. *Minimization.* You deny that things are an issue when they are: *You say "It's not a big deal!" (when it really is) or "I don't care!" (when you really do).*

9. **"Shoulding."** You have judgmental attitudes toward yourself and others: *"He shouldn't be so upset about it"* or *"I should be smarter and thinner than I am."*
10. **Making comparisons.** You compare yourself to others: *"He is so much smarter than me. I'm stupid."*
11. **Mental filter.** You focus on one negative detail and not the whole picture, discounting the positives: *"My large nose makes me look ugly."*
12. **Emotional reasoning.** If you feel it, you think it must be true: *"I feel like an idiot; therefore, I am."*
13. **Globalizing.** You see temporary feelings as permanent: *"I feel bad now, and always will."*

Handout 8.4: My Thoughts/Feelings/Behavior Log

This thoughts/feelings/behavior log will help you separate your thoughts, feelings, and behaviors, helping you identify faulty beliefs that result in negative consequences.

By replacing your negative thoughts with healthier ones, your feelings and behaviors will improve.

	Negative Beliefs, with % of certainty	Resulting Feelings	Resulting Behaviors	Alternative Rational Thoughts, with % of certainty	Resulting Feelings	Resulting Behaviors
1						
2						
3						
4						
5						

Handout 8.5: Self-Esteem Log

	Irrational Thoughts About Myself	Certainty of Beliefs (%)	Types of Cognitive Distortion	Alternative Rational Thoughts About Myself	Certainty of Beliefs (%)	Action Plan and Goals
1						
2						
3						
4						
5						

Sample Types of Faulty-Thinking Habits

1. **CATASTROPHIZING.** You label things as horrible and awful instead of unfortunate or disappointing: *"This is HORRIBLE!"*
2. **FORTUNE TELLING.** You think you can predict the future: *"I'll never find anyone who will be interested in me. I'll be alone the rest of my life."*
3. **BLACK-AND-WHITE THINKING.** You make all-or-nothing assumptions: *"All men are bad."*

4. **PERSONALIZATION.** You blame yourself for things that are out of your control: *"I am to blame for my child's issues."*
5. **JUMPING TO CONCLUSIONS.** You make assumptions and regard them as fact: *"He told me he can't come to the party. I bet he just doesn't like me."*
6. **LABELING.** You label yourself and others instead of being specific. Instead of saying, *"I made a mistake,"* you label yourself a *"failure"* or a *"loser."*
7. **MAGNIFICATION.** You make mountains out of molehills: *"This is the worst day of my life."*
8. **MINIMIZATION.** You deny that things are an issue when they are: *"It's not a big deal"* (when it really is) or *"I don't care"* (when you really do).
9. **"SHOULDING."** You have a judgmental attitude toward yourself and others: *"He shouldn't be so upset about it"* or *"I should be smarter and thinner."*
10. **MAKING COMPARISONS.** You compare yourself to others: *"He is so much smarter than me."*
11. **MENTAL FILTER.** You focus on one negative detail and not the whole picture, discounting the positives: *"I am ugly because of my large nose."*

By identifying thoughts that erode your self-esteem and pinpointing your erroneous thoughts and replacing them with healthier ones, you can devise an action plan for a better life.

Handout 8.6: My Weekly Self-Esteem Log

Date(s): _____

1. Upsetting thoughts about myself:

_____

2. Emotional responses:

_____

3. Degree of depressed feeling: LOW 1 2 3 4 5 6 7 8 9 10 HIGH

4. My behavioral reactions:

_____

5. Healthier thoughts about myself:

_____

   Degree of certainty: LOW 1 2 3 4 5 6 7 8 9 10 HIGH

6. CBT skills I have used this week:

_____

7. Mindfulness and acceptance skills I have practiced:

_____

8. Exercises and visualizations I have done:

_____

9. Costs and benefits of my low self-esteem:

_____

10. Action plan and goals for boosting my self-esteem:

_____

Recommended Resources

Self-Help Books

When Do the Good Things Start?
Abraham J. Twerski
Ten Days to Self-Esteem
David D. Burns

Clinician Books:

Cognitive Behavior Therapy: Basics and Beyond
Judith S. Beck
Ten Days to Self-Esteem: The Leader's Manual
(See especially "Double Standard Technique" and "Externalization of Voices," pp. 122–123)
David D. Burns

Links

Association for Contextual Behavioral Science
"Acceptance & Commitment Therapy (ACT)"
http://contextualscience.org/act
Beck Institute for Cognitive Therapy and Research
http://www.beckinstitute.org
Beck Institute Blog
http://www.beckinstituteblog.org
"50 Ways to Untwist Your Thinking" by David D. Burns
http://www.lauralcjohnson.com/uploads/50_Ways_to_Untwist_Your_Thinking_table__March_2005.pdf
Feeling Good: The Website of David D. Burns, MD
http://feelinggood.com
(David Burns's blog for therapists)
http://feelinggood.com/category/dr-davids-blogs/therapists-blog/
(Steven Hayes's website)
http://www.stevenchayes.com
The Linehan Institute: Behavioral Tech
(Marsha Linehan's DBT site)

http://behavioraltech.org

Psychology Tools

(CBT logs and forms)

http://www.psychologytools.org

Sources of Insight

"How To Use the Triple Column Technique to Defeat Negative Self-Talk"
http://sourcesofinsight.com/how-to-use-the-triple-column-technique/

CHAPTER NINE

The Regret Solution
Moving Past Remorse

Reworking the past never works. But that doesn't mean that our clients ever give up trying. Maybe it's because there's just too much hurt and pain involved, and they just can't "get over it." Some of our clients live life at an impasse, being too emotionally crippled to move forward and too emotionally crippled to leave the past behind before it's all figured out. Yet there comes a point when our clients need to make peace with their past, or they will be unable to make peace with their present. Not everything gets tied up in a neat package and bow. Life can be messy and untidy. We need to give our clients the tools they need to leave the past behind, even if they do not have the closure that they had hoped they would. Ruminating over past events rarely benefits our clients.

There are abundant opportunities to look back and rethink past decisions, with the notion that, given the chance to do it all over, things would be different. Most of our clients, like most people, have no shortage of regrets. Regrets in themselves are not to be avoided in life; rather, they guide us to make different decisions based on the wisdom we have learned from our experiences. However, regret can be painful. It is a very powerful emotion that can rob our clients of mental clarity and inner peace if they get stuck in the lands of "what might have been." Once today arrives, it becomes too late to live in yesterday, but some of our clients end up spending more time second-guessing yesterday than they do focusing on today. In fact, one of the most common goals that clients often have starting therapy is to find out "Why?"

Spending more time second-guessing yesterday unleashes powerful emotions that often keep our clients stuck, as they think if they found the keys to what went wrong, they can make things right in their lives. However, rarely does this type of uncovering lead to enlightenment or joy, and in fact, too much focus on making sense of the past without figuring out how to cope with life right now keeps our clients stuck in the past filled with regrets that have no hope of changing. After all, the past is past and it can not be changed. Only our take on the past and how we cope can really change. There is certainly a place in treatment for looking back, but teaching our clients new perspectives and life skills in coping with what happened will help them turn regrets and past misfortunes to wiser decisions at present, serving as a motivator rather than a detractor of psychological well-being. However, it is true that using regret as a motivator is not an easy nut to crack with our clients, as regret most often serves instead as a barrier to healing and personal growth. Perhaps regret is so tough because regret leads to self-blame, and a basic sense in our clients that they somehow have failed.

One of the best gifts we can give to our clients steeped in regret is to focus on growth. Unconditional acceptance and assurance that they are still good people despite their human failings is reassuring. As we saw in the last chapter on self-esteem, clients will be unable to move forward unless they feel safe and accepted in the therapeutic relationship. Likewise, patience and non-judgmentalness can set the stage for overcoming regret. Clients are already often mad enough at themselves already, figuratively kicking themselves for things they said and did that they can't take back. Unconditional acceptance from the therapist will set the stage for them to heal and move forward in the therapeutic relationship, rather than spending their lives looking into the rearview mirror.

Due to the immobilizing effects of self-blame and shame, implicit in the quest for overcoming regret is the need for our clients to work on self-forgiveness (see Chapter 7). Sometimes we also need to encourage our clients to ask for forgiveness from others whom they believe that they have hurt. Often a vital part of overcoming regret is taking constructive action at present. At times, the very act of asking for forgiveness can be a pivotal point in overcoming regret and growing from it. Most often, a sincere act of remorse and acceptance of responsibility will help clients get some amount of support from others, even from those who were wronged. However, even without a favorable response from others, or in the absence of that opportunity for interaction, expressing remorse in therapy sessions through role-play can be beneficial. Therapists can help clients achieve some sense of self-forgiveness with support and empathy, helping them realize that they did the best they could with what they knew and were capable of at the time. After all, we can urge our clients to stop expecting themselves to be able to give themselves and others what they did not have themselves to give at the time. It's easy to have 20/20 hindsight as a Monday morning quarterback. Furthermore, reminding your clients that just as they can't expect to buy milk at a furniture store, they might take comfort in the fact that they couldn't handle situations differently if they lacked the skills and knowledge to do so back then. I encourage my clients to focus on what they learned from the past rather than on living in it. After all, they have a choice: Live in the past, or learn from it!

As with most emotional reactions, there is a continuum of regret, from normal and mild regret that offers life lessons moving forward to debilitating regret that leads to emotional paralysis and depression. The simple words "If only," "I wish," or "I should have" all have the potential to provide our clients with pangs of guilt that can end up being a life sentence of looking through the rearview mirror. Our role as therapists is to help our clients get past the land of "woulda coulda shoulda."

Cognitive Behavior Therapy (CBT) psychologist and author Arthur Freeman addresses the regretful words that became the title of his book *Woulda, Coulda, Shoulda* (1989). His use of CBT helps clients unblock themselves from being overwhelmed with regrets from the past, and offers hope that it's never too late to move past the "woulda, coulda, shoulda" thinking that continues to plague individuals, robbing them of inner peace and life satisfaction. As Freeman wrote, "There is no shortage of mines to step on. There is no shortage of ways to 'go wrong.'"

Freeman does admit that there is a place in everyone's life to review their choices and even mistakes, and reflect on how things could be different moving forward. Revisiting has its place in helping us learn and grow stronger, but just like daily vitamins can be toxic if we take too many in a day, spending time steeped in regret will be toxic for our mental health. After all, we don't get "do-overs" in life. When our clients ruminate, it permeates everything they experience in life. Their every day is tainted with a gnawing sense that something went wrong, and people spend hours, days, weeks, months, and even years second-guessing themselves and trying to make peace with their past.

For example, 38-year-old Daniel spent most of his life regretting that he had been short-tempered and verbally abusive to his ex-girlfriend. After years of enduring his anger and temper, she left him and eventually got married and had a family. Even though it had been more than eight years, Daniel could not forgive himself and could not seem to find another woman to replace her. He lived with guilt and could not stop thinking about how he had "screwed up." He felt alone and hopeless and spent way too much of his free time ruminating about how he'd lost his best chance for a happy life, living in guilt and regret. He also regretted that he had partied too much in college and dropped out as a sopho-more, and now he felt like he was in a dead end job. In essence, he was a prisoner of his "woulda, coulda, shouldas." Daniel kept questioning why he was so clueless, and why he acted the way he did. I emphasized to him that focusing on the "whys" is actually not wise, as he would really never know for sure and would just keep on going in circles trying to figure our something that could never be fully figured out. Sometimes the best we can do with our clients is to help them shift to "what's next?"

In the following treatment tips section, I offer the practical solutions I used with Daniel and clients like him, as well as other solutions to the very common problem of regret.

Treatment Tips

☑ CBT Technique: Help Clients Identify
Common Thinking Errors

As shown in previous chapters, one of the hallmarks of CBT interven-tion is helping clients identify their cognitive distortions. I have used cognitive distortion lists in various handouts in other chapters of this book, as this cornerstone of CBT is essential to effective treatment for every type of client problem. When my clients and I examine their irra-tional thoughts, I often use a handout with a list of cognitive distortions to help them identify the types of faulty thinking they are using. In the case of Daniel, I used this type of handout, containing a description of the common thinking errors listed below, to help him identify his cognitive error habits. Identifying cognitive distortions is a great step toward limiting ruminative regrets.

Common Thinking Errors

ALL-OR-NOTHING THINKING. You see things in black-or-white categories. If you make a mistake, you might think that you "failed" and or are a "failure."

MIND READING. You make assumptions that people are doing something to you on purpose, or you jump to conclusions and treat attributions that are opinion as fact.

BLAMING. You feel like a victim and believe that others are at fault for your feelings and reactions.

OVERGENERALIZATION. You generalize from a specific. You think in absolutes, like "always" and "never," and see a single negative event as a never-ending pattern.

BLOWING THINGS OUT OF PROPORTION. You make rigid assumptions that lead to all-or-nothing thinking and blow things out of proportion.

MENTAL FILTER. You pick out a negative single event and dwell on it, like a drop of ink that discolors a whole beaker of water.

MINIMIZATION. You deny that something is a problem when it is, rationalizing "It's not such a big deal" when it really is.

"SHOULD" STATEMENTS. You have preconceived ideas of how you and other people "should" be. Judgmental and unforgiving expectations create a lot of anxiety and anger.

PERSONALIZATION. You are self-conscious and think things are about you when that is just your interpretation. You think that if someone is negative, it is in response to you, and then blame yourself.

MAKING COMPARISONS. You compare yourself to others and feel inferior.

FORTUNE TELLING. You think that you can predict the future and convince yourself that bad things will happen.

LABELING. You label yourself or others by terms such as "lazy," "fat," "stupid," "loser," and "jerk," stating them as facts. A label becomes an erroneous evaluation of personal worth.

SELECTIVE or EMOTIONAL REASONING. You take things out of context, jumping to conclusions while disregarding other information.

☑ Activity: Have Your Client Write Their Regrets

After my clients look at the cognitive distortions list, I have them write down their regrets for homework, or we compile a list in the session, and use the list to identify their distortions.

In his book, Freeman (1989) emphasizes the importance of having clients write their regrets down. Going back to the example above, I had Daniel write down for homework the specific thoughts of ruminative regret that were destroying his life. This is what his assignment looked like:

I never should have mistreated her.
I should have known better.
I'll never find anyone like her.
I'm miserable and I will never be happy.
I blew my one shot for happiness in life.

In reviewing the homework, I asked Daniel what he noticed about his list. He noticed that it was all negative and irrational, but he claimed he really believed it, and how could he change something he really believed? I was glad to have handouts such as "Common Thinking Errors" (Handout 9.2) in my therapeutic toolbox to help him find out for himself why these thoughts were not true. Other handouts that might be helpful to assign your clients between sessions so that they can process their regret are "My Regret Log" (Handout 9.5) and the "Weekly Summary Log for Overcoming Regret" (Handout 9.6).

In session, I helped Daniel identify the type of cognitive distortion for each of the items on his list and kept this sheet as a model for further self-help assignments. This is what it looked like:

Regret Self-Talk	Type of Cognitive Error
I should have known better— *I'm an idiot.*	Labeling, "should" statement
I'll never find anyone like her.	Fortune telling, overgeneralization
I'm miserable and I will never *be happy.*	Fortune telling, all-or-nothing thinking
I blew my one shot for happiness *in life.*	All-or-nothing thinking, emotional reasoning
I'm such a loser—I'm the worst in *the family.*	Labeling, making comparisons, magnification
Why was I such an insensitive fool?	Labeling, blaming, catastrophizing

As you can see, Daniel was still stuck in the "whys" of his life. He ruminated about what went wrong, trying to find the pieces to the puzzle. However, rarely can we help our clients get a definitive answer on why things went wrong. It's all a matter of conjecture and keeps the conversation focused on the past. When our clients spend too much time in the land of "Why?" it's helpful to shift their focus to "What's next?"

☑ *Mini-Lesson: Help Clients Shift From "Why?"* *to "What's Next?"*

To help clients overcome regret and shift from "Why?" to "What's next?" I ask them to brainstorm with me a list of their "whys," and I write them down. I then ask them to rephrase each "why" into a "what's next" question. "What's next?" becomes a type of plan. It is oriented to something clients can do today based on their past regrets. In other words, it is a call to action.

Using Daniel's question "Why was I such an insensitive fool?" the "what's next" alternative could be "I have learned a lot in that relationship and will be sure to put that knowledge in my next relationship. Although I wish I knew then what I know now, I apparently had some growing up to do and did not have the maturity until recently. I need to accept that it is just part of being human. I will work on now accepting myself as a flawed human being, and work on enjoying life instead of berating myself. I deserve it."

The "why" questions we have in everyday life can also be replaced with a "what's next" attitude, as we really will never know *why* things are—we can only conjecture.

Here are some examples. Instead of asking "Why is my coworker acting so rude?" a client might say, "When he acts rudely, I will tell him I will not continue our discussion until he addresses me more respectfully." Instead of asking, "Why am I so sensitive?" a client might say, "I tend to be shy when speaking in groups. To help me with this tendency, I will write down my negative thoughts that make me anxious and work on replacing them with healthier ones."

☑ Mini-Lesson: Help Clients Turn Unproductive Regret to Productive Regret

Psychologist and author Neal Roese (2005) shows us that regret is universal. He spent more than a decade doing research on regret and found four main areas of regret that many of us share:

1. Regrets about education
2. Career regrets
3. Regrets in love
4. Parenting regrets

It does seem that my clients' regrets often fall in one of these four categories. Clients are often dissatisfied with their jobs, wishing they had gotten more education. Others wish they had never gotten married to the wrong person and wonder what would have happened and how life could have been different if they got to choose over again with what they know now. Others are parents whose children did not turn out as they had hoped, and look for clues of where they went wrong in raising them. In these cases, there is very little solace or comfort in reasoning "you did the best you could," because they cling to the notion that they should have known better, even if they didn't, and they just can't forgive themselves for not knowing then what they know now.

It is important to note with your clients that the term *regret* carries the implicit notion that they are in fact to blame, and therefore guilt weighs on them heavily. Often our clients take on more of the lion's share of responsibility and blame when in fact it is often really very little about them at all. Perhaps the most important thing we can do for a client struggling with regret is to help them forgive themselves for not having the foresight into what is now so obvious in hindsight. After all, life is a learning curve, and we can't expect ourselves to have known everything since we were seven!

These are some points to make with your clients about turning unproductive regrets into productive regrets:

1. Regrets are important in our life to help us self-correct. The key is to recover from and build on the sharp sting of regret to look for lessons learned and take comfort in the fact that these lessons make us wiser.
2. Take comfort in the fact that regrets help us develop empathy for others. Empathy is considered to be one of the cornerstones of emotional intelligence.
3. The more wrong turns you made in retrospect, the more you increase the odds that your future choices will be more prudent.
4. Having learned so many lessons from mistakes or regrets, you will be in better shape moving forward.
5. No one tries to be toxic or dysfunctional. People generally try their best, even if their best is not objectively healthy. Unhealthy people make unhealthy decisions and behave in an unhealthy way. People do not intentionally make self-defeating decisions.
6. A lack of forgiveness for oneself or others is one of the most common reasons for depression, anxiety, and interpersonal conflict. Thankfully, regrets give you the opportunity to self-correct and to develop the ability to forgive. Strive to be thankful

for this golden opportunity to release yourself from bitterness and negativity for good!

7. Use the broken pieces of unrealized dreams and disappointments as stepping-stones toward a better future.

8. You cannot change what happened to you, but you can change what you do with what happened to you.

Dale Carnegie (1948) wrote, "You can't saw sawdust," and told of the time he was in high school and his science teacher offered one of the most memorable and profound lessons in his early schooling. His teacher had his students crowd around his lab sink and push over a bottle of milk while crying out, "No use crying over spilt milk!"

☑ *Activity: Helping Clients Move From Guilt To Gratitude*
What do these simple phrases have in common?

I should have . . .
I shouldn't have . . .
I could have . . .
If only I . . .
I can't believe I . . .
Why didn't I . . .

Some degree of guilt is good for you and necessary in making you into a person who learns from mistakes. But guilt often distorts perceptions and is based on mistakes and errors that were not quite as terrible as your clients thought, or that never really happened.

Below are some examples of how to help clients change their self-talk. Similar to the previous section on moving from "why" to "what's next," this section on moving from guilt to gratitude will be useful in helping your clients keep themselves from starting their thoughts with these phrases that are filled with judgment and shame.

"Going from Guilt to Gratitude" (Handout 9.4) offers you and your clients another opportunity to transform their negative regret into positive regret, as the present becomes the focus instead of the stagnant past.

The handout is blank, so here are some examples you could offer your client before they fill out the sheet between sessions.

Guilt Statement	Gratitude Statement
I shouldn't have <u>raised my voice at him.</u>	I am grateful that I <u>have the chance to "make it right."</u>
I should have <u>known better.</u>	I am grateful that I <u>know better now.</u>
I could have <u>done better.</u>	I am grateful that I <u>can try to do better now.</u>
If only <u>I had made better choices,</u>	I am grateful that I <u>can I use my life lessons as a springboard for other choices.</u>
I could have <u>been so much better off with him.</u>	I am grateful that I <u>learned good lessons to improve present and future relationships.</u>
If only I <u>went to college.</u>	I am grateful that <u>it's not too late.</u>
I can't believe I <u>acted like an idiot.</u>	I am grateful that I <u>am a work in progress.</u>

☑ CBT Technique: "Should" Busting—in a Jar

For homework or in the session, have your clients compose a written "should" list. Have them write sentences that start with "I should have" and then replace the "should" messages with more self-compassionate ones. For example, "I should never have treated him like that" can be replaced with, "If I was healthier at the time, I would not have treated him like that." Replacing the "shoulds" with more rational thoughts will help your clients learn from them rather than being stuck in them.

You might want to give your clients the rule that "shoulding" on themselves is not permitted. In my office, I actually have a "should" jar, and I often point to this jar when clients "should" on themselves. There are times that I have had clients bring in "should" notes from home or write them during the session, then put them in the jar—and out of their heads!

At home, clients can create their own " should jar," affixing the word *should* on an empty jar. Then, on note cards, they can write negative "should" messages that come to mind, and put it out of their head and into the jar. Symbolically, this jar helps clients release themselves from their inner critic putting their "shoulds" out of their heads.

☑ Activity: Write a Self-Forgiveness Letter

Clients who are steeped in regret are stuck by an inability to forgive themselves. Sometimes it helps clients to write a letter to their earlier selves, the younger self that meant well but fell short. When clients write a letter to this younger version of themselves, encourage them to show compassion to their younger selves, reminding them that their earlier self deserves a good life, despite being human and flawed. This is a nice exercise in self-compassion.

☑ Activity: Self-Compassion

In this exercise, have your clients think of some affirmations for themselves and write them down. Suggest that they remind themselves of these affirmations daily. One client used these very powerful words: "I am worthy. I am a good person. I deserve to be happy, and I will choose today to be happy and enjoy my life now."

Instruct your clients to look at themselves in the mirror every morning and repeat their chosen affirmations. Rather than looking at themselves from inside their heads, they can use a mirror in this exercise to help them look at themselves from the outside as they watch themselves saying the encouraging words to themselves. Suggestion: To experience the effectiveness of doing this, put down this book now and try it yourself!

☑ DBT Activity: Growing Through Distress

Have your clients take a moment to describe a regret that is currently haunting them. Then, write one fiction and one fact takeaway, as you see below.

Regret:

"I regret I did not take that job"

Fiction:

"I would be happier working there than at my present job."

"I was so unrealistic—I should have known better."

Facts:

"I made the best decision I could at the time, and I don't know how other choices would have turned out."

"I will use this disappointment as an opportunity to reevaluate my life and make different decisions now—including looking for another job."

In helping clients accept their regrets and stop fighting them, Dialectical Behavior Therapy (DBT) founder Marsha Linehan uses the acronym ACCEPTS as a distress tolerance skill for warding off intense feelings of upset. The acronym is meant to remind people of the important skills that they need to practice to tolerate distress. It can offer an action plan for accepting the pangs of regret and moving on past it. It is basically an action plan for when the emotional distress is too persistent. It is usually carried out in the context of what Linehan calls WISE MIND ACCEPTS, which means that when your figurative *emotional mind* works in conjunction with your figurative *logical mind* perspective, that is where wisdom is found. The following acronym, representing a cluster of skills recommended for living a healthier life, is an example of an item on a DBT diary log that is regularly used.

Activities: Engage in activities you enjoy.

Contributing: Help others, volunteer, give of yourself.

Comparisons: Compare yourself with others who are also struggling, and it will help you realize you are not alone.

Emotions: Find an activity to bring out different emotions, such as music, a TV show, taking a walk, reading a joke book, and so forth.

Push: Push away the situation, or in this case, push away the regret. Visualize putting it into a box or on a shelf.

Thoughts: Replace with non-emotional thoughts, such as counting to 10, thinking about a game or puzzle on your phone, etc.

Sensation: Focus on opposing sensations, such as holding an ice cube or squeezing a stress ball.

☑ Activity: Use Metaphors and Visualizations to Help Clients Heal Regret

Below are a few metaphors for regret:

The hungry tiger. One of the best-known metaphoric stories from ACT founder Steven Hayes is that of the hungry tiger. In his parable, he refers to a figurative tiger that grows as it is being fed red meat, just as our regrets and negative thoughts grow when we feed them. His thought is that the more you resist being aware of painful thoughts and emotions, the more you feed the hungry tiger. When you resist the pain of regret, you are actually feeding the tiger more meat, and he becomes more powerful. Every time you practice avoidance, you feed the beast and lose more control over your life.

Rear-view mirror visualization. This is an excellent visualization for helping your clients imagine what will happen if they look backward instead of forward in life, and the perils of living in the past rather than in the present. A rearview mirror is a powerful metaphor for illustrating the absurdity of trying to move forward while looking backward. If you were actually on the road, it wouldn't take too long to get into an accident!

Ruminative "chewing" metaphors. Mulling over your regrets is like chewing a piece of gum over and over—it ends up losing its flavor. Sure, it may taste fresh at the beginning, but the more you chew it—just as the more you concentrate on the regrets in your life—the more and flavor—or vitality—they lose. It might be interesting to educate your clients about the origins of the word *rumination.* It is taken from the Latin word *ruminari,* meaning to chew the cud. This word is taken from the behavior of a cow, who brings up and chews the same food again and swallows it again; it keeps going to another of the cow's four stomachs to facilitate digestion. The cow chewing its cud is a great visualization for rumination, meaning one who chews, regurgitates, and rechews the same food over and over again. The difference between humans and cows, of course, is that cows need to "ruminate" to get nutrients for their survival because they eat hard-to-digest foods, and they chew their cud about eight hours a day. People, on the other hand, tend to chew on the same thoughts over and over during most of their waking hours, robbing them of their mental health. I find that using real-life metaphors such as these helps clients make the connection to their own lives and helps motivate them to make life changes.

The Swiss cheese metaphor. My own personal favorite metaphor is the premise of *The Swiss Cheese Theory of Life* (Belmont & Shor, 2012). Swiss cheese reminds us that we all have holes in our lives, and to expect life to be smooth and predictable like cream cheese or American cheese is unrealistic. Rather, the distinctiveness of the Swiss cheese is a result of its holes, and the key to resiliency is to find ways to bounce back from adversity and get through life's holes without getting stuck in them. When we order Swiss at the deli counter, we expect it to have holes. Why not see your life that way?

Acknowledging the inevitability of regret is the one way to make peace and move on from it. To further the Swiss cheese analogy, the bigger the holes, the more flavorful the cheese—just as in our lives, overcoming challenges is how we develop character; we too become more distinctive!

Thus, regrets can actually help us develop our insight and character. After all, would you really want to be bland and predictable like American cheese or cream cheese?

☑ Activity: Transform Regrets Into Goals

One of my favorite tips for helping clients overcome regret is to put a positive spin on regret by transforming regrets into a call to action. It starts with focusing on a regret that they have, and then asking them to transform it into a goal.

Below is an example:

Regret: I should have spent more time enjoying my kids when they were young instead of working so hard.

Goal: I will put more effort into forging a better relationship with them now, putting them before my work.

By focusing on proactive action instead of what can never be changed, you will give your client a gift of a second chance. One of my favorite sayings is, "There are no do-overs, but there are second chances!"

☑ ACT Mindfulness Visualizations: Overcoming Regret

Mindfulness and acceptance practices are a major component of third-wave approaches such as DBT, Acceptance and Commitment Therapy (ACT), and Mindfulness-Based Cognitive Therapy (MBCT). The term *mindfulness* doesn't necessarily mean being in a meditative state with your eyes closed. Rather, it is a nonjudgmental awareness in everyday life, in which one is present and focused but without judgment. It has been called having a "Teflon mind" to which thoughts do not stick. Regrets, worries, sad thoughts come and go and don't get caught in the mental web of past regret or future worry.

One of the main premises of Acceptance and Commitment Therapy is acceptance of the inevitable pain of being human, and living life in the present and to the fullest despite it. Rather than fighting the pain, clients use the principles of ACT to flow with the current and experience the pain of regret rather than trying to make it go away. DBT founder Linehan calls present centeredness without judgment *radical acceptance*, which mean total acceptance without fighting thoughts and feelings, watching letting them come and go without judgment. With your clients, visualizations and metaphors for mindfulness can be helpful. You might want to use the metaphor of a river, having your clients imagine that they are on a riverbank, watching all their regrets and negative thoughts float by, instead of being in there swimming and immersed in that way of thinking.

Another nice metaphor from ACT founder Hayes is "tug of war with a monster." In this metaphor, imagine there is a bottomless pit between you and the monster, and that the more you tug, the closer you get to the pit. The best thing for avoiding falling into the pit is to let go, which is a symbol of not fighting anymore but accepting the thoughts that cause the figurative tug of war.

A Toolkit of Metaphors for Overcoming Regret

For individuals struggling with regret, assembling items for a regret-busting metaphorical toolkit will help remind them of the importance of healing from regret. Following are some of the items that serve as great metaphors for your clients regret-busting toolkit.

> **An eraser.** It's okay to make mistakes. Regrets are a result of not being perfect. After all, we are not born with a blueprint for having the foresight to know what we now know in hindsight!
>
> **A Band-Aid.** This reminds us to heal our wounds with forgiveness, giving us the chance to soothe ourselves with healing thoughts and to free ourselves from self-recriminating thoughts of regret.
>
> **Dice.** Life is a game of chance—you never know how things are going to work out, and you play the game as best you can.
>
> **Deck of cards.** Each of us is given a hand in life, but it's up to us to play that hand. If we feel like we're losing the game, we can reshuffle and play again. We might not have a full deck of cards, but we play with what we have!
>
> **Magnifying glass.** Look closely to identify cognitive distortions.
>
> **Toy cow.** Cows chew their cud over and over again to digest the grass in a process called *ruminari*, which is the origin of the word *ruminate*. (You can often find bags of farm animals at the dollar store.)
>
> **Chewing gum.** Chewing gum over and over again until it loses its flavor is like what happens when we chew over the past.

Can you and your clients think of other metaphors for regret?

Therapeutic Takeaways

☑ Help your clients recognize attitudes that can help them move from unproductive regret to productive regret.

☑ Help clients identify the common cognitive distortions that result in ruminative regret.

☑ Writing activities for overcoming regret, such as self-forgiveness letters or identifying the cognitive distortions behind regrets, can be very helpful for clients between and within sessions.

☑ With a healthier perspective, guilt can be replaced by gratitude.

☑ Help your clients to identity the common cognitive errors that result in guilt.

☑ Help your clients move from asking "Why?" to asking "What's next?"

☑ Using metaphors can help clients move on from regret.

Handouts

The following worksheets will help your clients to overcome regret. These worksheets have been referred to in the body of this chapter. As a general guideline, handouts and assignments are given to clients at the end of the session. Make sure you leave ample time to go over your expectations for use of the selected handouts.

When assignments are given out, it is important to follow up with your clients at the beginning of the next session by going over their homework with them. Going over homework is an essential aspect of being a solution-oriented therapist.

Note: All handouts in the book are available for download on my website by following the link below: http://www.belmontwellness.com/ultimate-solution-handouts/

Handout 9.1: Common Myths About Regret

Myth 1: Regret is bad and unproductive in our lives.

To the contrary, regret (within reason) is a very important psychological reaction we have as humans, and it helps us to be productive members of society. In fact, one of the hallmarks of people with antisocial personality disorders, who populate our prisons, is the absence of regret and a tendency to blame others while not learning from mistakes.

Thus, we need regret in order to take responsibility for wrongful actions and to do better in the future. The problem comes when regret is extreme and debilitating, robbing us of self-esteem and well-being. It exists on a continuum, but a healthy degree of regret is vital to a well-functioning life. The key is to have your regret work to improve you rather than hinder you.

Myth 2: Regret is rarely productive.

Regret can be divided into two categories: productive regret and unproductive regret. Unproductive regret leads to self-berating and emotional paralysis due to an all-pervasive "I-should-have-known-better" attitude.

The problem is that you can't change the past, and what's done is done. The best way to move past this no-win situation is to use lessons learned to make the regret productive, using it as a springboard for making better choices going forward. One of the greatest stings in life is that of regret, and by turning that sting into improved insight and action, we can actually increase our self-esteem instead of diminishing it.

Myth 3: Regret and Guilt are interchangeable.

Although they can often be intertwined, there is a very definite difference between guilt and regret. Regret can be quite healthy and is what's behind the words "I'm sorry." Taking responsibility for words you wish you didn't say or actions you wish you didn't do is a normal human reaction and necessary for character building and growth.

Guilt, however, runs deeper and tends to be less objective and rational. It entails a sense of shame and is much more emotionally intense and harder to move past. It robs us of self-esteem and a sense of self-worth, and is often caught up in our imagination. While regret is generally felt for past actions that are regarded as forgivable, guilt is typically steeped in unresolved internal shame-based perceptions that rarely pass the test of objective reality.

The word *remorse* comes from the Latin word meaning "to bite again" and is a deep form of guilt that causes people to keep hurting themselves. Whereas regret can be a response of mild disappointment, remorse over a "wrong" or a regrettable action weighs heavily on the heart and mind.

Myth 4: Regret is mostly about wrong paths taken.

Although regret is often a reaction to our words and actions, many times regret is actually a reaction to a nonaction and a road not taken:

"I wish I had worked harder in school."

"I wish I had gone into another profession."

"I wish I'd made more friends when I was in college."

"I wish I had gotten married."

"I wish I had never gotten married."

"I wish I was more appreciative of the freedom I had when I was younger."

"I wish I told her how much I loved her when I had the chance."

These are examples of regrets of inaction. Neal Roese, in his book *If Only: How to Turn Regret Into Opportunity* (2005), writes about the inevitability that most of us will spend at least some time thinking about "what might have been" and urges his readers to use this information as a guide to changing their present life. He also regards regret as a great motivator to look for "opportunities knocking" in the present, while pointing out that regret is one the greatest propellers of action and can help motivate us to be more proactive in our lives *now*.

Handout 9.2: Common Thinking Errors

1. *ALL-OR-NOTHING THINKING:* You see things in black-and-white categories. If you make a mistake, you might think that you "failed" or are a "failure."
2. *OVERGENERALIZATION:* You generalize from a specific. You think in absolutes, like *always* and *never*, and see a single negative event as a never-ending pattern.
3. *MENTAL FILTER:* You pick out a single negative event and dwell on it, like a drop of ink that discolors a whole glass of water.
4. *MAGNIFICATION or MINIMIZATION:* You either blow things out of proportion or deny that something is a problem when it is. Examples: *"I am the worst mother ever"* or *"It's nothing—no big deal"* (when it really is a big deal to you).
5. *"SHOULD" STATEMENTS:* You have preconceived ideas about how you and other people "should" be. Judgmental and unforgiving expectations create a lot of anxiety.
6. *PERSONALIZATION:* You are self-conscious and think things are about you when that is just your interpretation. When someone behaves negatively, you think that that behavior is a response to you, and then blame yourself.
7. *PLAYING THE COMPARISON GAME:* You compare yourself to others and feel the need to keep up with or outshine others to feel good about yourself. Example: "He is so much smarter than me; I'm stupid."
8. *FORTUNE TELLING:* You think that you can predict the future, and you convince yourself that bad things will happen. Example: "I will always have these problems!"
9. *LABELING:* You label yourself or others by terms such as *lazy, fat, stupid, loser,* and *jerk,* stating them as if they were facts. A label becomes an erroneous evaluation of self-worth.
10. *SELECTIVE or EMOTIONAL REASONING:* You take things out of context, jumping to conclusions while disregarding the other information. For example, a client claimed she was just like her estranged mother because she looked like her, although she listed many other ways that they were not alike.

Handout 9.3: Transforming Unproductive Regret to Productive Regret

Yes, regret can be productive!

We can choose whether to learn from the past or to lament it. If regret robs you of happiness and life satisfaction, this worksheet can help you move past unproductive regret to productive regret.

Below, write down some of the unproductive regrets that hold you back in your life, and transform them into productive regrets. Make them a call for action.

Unproductive Regret	Productive Regret
Example: I regret my insensitivity to what my family needed from me.	I will work on being kinder and less judgmental toward my family and others in my life now. I will use these regrets to better myself.

Handout 9.4: Going From Guilt to Gratitude

Fill in the blanks, transforming the guilt-producing thoughts into kinder thoughts that lead to gratitude rather than guilt.

Guilt Statement   **Gratitude Statement**

I shouldn't have taken this job.   I am grateful that I have a job and can look into finding another.

I should have _____   I am grateful that I _____
_____   _____

I could have _____   I am grateful that I _____
_____   _____

If only I _____   I am grateful that I _____
_____   _____

I could have _____   I am grateful that I _____
_____   _____

If only I had _____   I am grateful that I _____
_____   _____

I can't believe I _____   I still have the opportunity to _____
_____   _____

Why couldn't I have _____   I am grateful that I _____
_____   _____

Why didn't I _____   I am grateful that I _____
_____   _____

Handout 9.5: My Regret Log

For this log, think of a situation in which you were consumed with regret.

My Regret
Negative Emotions
Strength of Negative Emotions 1 2 3 4 5 6 7 8 9 10 Low   High
Identify Negative Beliefs Underlying the Regret
Type of Cognitive Distortion (Thinking Error)
Certainty of Your Beliefs 1 2 3 4 5 6 7 8 9 10 Low   High
Unhealthy Reactions in Response to the Regret
Cost/Benefit Analysis of Holding On to the Regret Costs: Benefits:

Handout 9.6: Weekly Summary Log For Overcoming Regret

Date(s): _____

1. My regret:

_____

2. Emotional responses:

_____

3. Degree of anxiety: LOW 1 2 3 4 5 6 7 8 9 10 HIGH

4. Unhealthy thoughts:

_____

    Degree of certainty: LOW 1 2 3 4 5 6 7 8 9 10 HIGH

5. Type of cognitive distortion:

_____

6. Healthy alternatives:

_____

    Certainty of beliefs: LOW 1 2 3 4 5 6 7 8 9 10 HIGH

7. Unhealthy reactions:

_____

8. Healthy reactions:

_____

9. Metaphors and visualizations I this week:

_____

10. Alternative skills I can use :

_____

11. Costs and benefits of my healthy and unhealthy thinking:

_____

12. Goal for improving my skills to overcome regret:

_____

Recommended Resources

Self-Help Books

Ten Days To Self-Esteem
  David D. Burns
Woulda, Coulda, Shoulda: Overcoming Regrets, Mistakes, and Missed
  Opportunities
  Arthur Freeman and Rose DeWolf
If Only: How to Turn Regret Into Opportunity
  Neal Roese

Links

AARP Bulletin

"Don't Let Regrets Ruin Your Health: How to Wise Up and Move On" by
  Dorothy Foltz-Gray
  http://www.aarp.org/health/healthy-living/info-03-2012/how-to
  -overcome-regrets-protect-health.html

Psych Central

"Got Regret? The Top 10 American Regrets" by John M. Grohol
  http://psychcentral.com/blog/archives/2011/03/24/got-regret-the
  -top-10-american-regrets/

Psychology Today

"Guilt"
  http://www.psychologytoday.com/basics/guilt
"Personal Growth: Woulda, Coulda, Shoulda: What Is the Worst Emotion You Could Experience?" by Jim Taylor
  http://www.psychologytoday.com/blog/the-power-prime/201205/
  personal-growth-woulda-coulda-shoulda
"The Psychology of Regret: Should We Live Our Lives With No Regrets
  as the Song Tells Us To?" by Melanie Greenberg
  http://www.psychologytoday.com/collections/201311/your-future
  -self/the-psychology-regret

CHAPTER TEN

The Change-Resistance Solution
Flexibility for Personal Transformation

It's not uncommon to hear clients say, "I don't like change." In fact, change resistance in clients is one of the most challenging issues that many therapists face. Just as our clients may have difficulty in changing their ingrained maladaptive habits in counseling, they also have often a hard time coping with the outward changes in their lives—even changes that are positive and actually sought after. Many clients express frustration, especially when change is sudden and unexpected and seemingly out of their control. The point I make with my clients is that change is like stress—it is an inevitable part of life and it is neither good nor bad; it just *is*.

Often we see that clients who have low self-esteem and basic insecurity have the hardest time adapting to change as well as making life changes. Adapting to change comes much easier for those who are more secure and feel less needy. In Dialectical Behavior Therapy (DBT), change impairment in clients denotes a lack of flexibility, such in the case of personality disorders, where they are stuck in a "survival mode" rather than a "change mode." The therapeutic approaches of the third wave of treatment address the needs of the change-resistant client when traditional cognitive treatment is not enough. DBT, Acceptance and Commitment Therapy (ACT), and Mindfulness-Based Cognitive Therapy (MBCT) are all examples of third-wave approaches that originated from the difficulty of traditional cognitive treatments to reach hard-to-treat clients, such as those with borderline personality disorder or other ingrained personality disorders. People with personality disorders are often shielded in rigid defend mechanisms that were adaptive in terms of survival during times of emotional upheaval in their past. Such clients often learn to compartmentalize their conflicting needs, thoughts, and behaviors, leading to poor coping skills and immature behavior.

Acceptance and mindfulness practices are important facets of effective third-wave approaches with treatment-resistant clients. Mindfulness and acceptance strategies help treatment-resistant clients accept the inevitability of some pain in their lives which helps them develop a more objective, mature, and detached awareness of their difficult emotions and thoughts. Rather than feeling immobilized by these emotions and thoughts and seeing things in absolutes (i.e., "I will *never* get over this" or "He is *bad* and I *hate* him"), our change-resistant clients can be taught ways to be more flexible in their perceptions. For example, in the act of cognitive defusion, which is a cornerstone of acceptance strategies, problematic thoughts and emotions are experienced indirectly by an "observing head" that looks *at* troubling emotions nonjudgmentally rather than looking *from* them. The phrase "Don't believe everything you think" is an example of a non-judgmental stance.

It is not surprising that clients with personality disorders are the ones who are the most change resistant. Since their "survival mode" results quite often from trauma early on, from an unstable or even abusive childhood to traumatic love relationships, clients come for counseling needing support and non-judgmental validation before they feel the safety net to make changes. Such clients come to therapy seeking a refuge of peace and security, often raw over the unpredictability of others in their lives and driven by the need for predictability and stability. Therapists and clients who are frustrated over the client's lack of progress in making major life changes may find third-wave strategies very effective in getting clients "unstuck."

For the change-resistant client, metaphors can also significantly unlock emotion and insight where mere talking cannot. Metaphors conjure up images that promote understanding. Imagine a tadpole turning into a frog. This demonstrates the idea of transformation more powerfully than just talking with your client about the need to grow and transform. How about a seed that transforms into a beautiful flower? On a more grand scale, how about an egg that turns into a chicken, or an acorn that turns into a tree? A chameleon transforms itself to adapt to its environment. Brainstorming examples of nature's transformations is a fun group exercise.

For those who say they don't like change, they are not considering the birth of a child or grandchild, making a new friend, going on vacation, getting a new job or promotion, winning a contest, or moving to a bigger house in a more desirable neighborhood. We would be hard pressed to find people who don't like those types of changes! Of course, with all desired changes, even the most desired ones, comes its new set of anxieties and stresses from going out of our comfort zone, such as fear of failure, leaving the safety of the old neighborhood to go to a new one, or leaving the security of your home and accustomed environs to travel to different parts of the state, country or even the world. Most of us have heard of the lottery winners who were unlucky enough to get their prayers answered, and winning the lottery led to personal setbacks and even family tragedy. Thus, with each change—even the most desired ones—comes its share of challenges and anxieties. Case in point— change is a mixed bag—and increasingly change resiliency and the ability to have control over our life changes will help to limit negative effects of life's inevitable changes.

Thus, change itself is not the problem; everyone wants to see their loved ones—and themselves—grow, evolve, and mature. What they generally see as problematic is change that they can't control, which leaves them feeling even more powerless.

It is our responsibility as therapists not only to help our clients by providing good listening skills, support, and guidance, but also to serve as life skills educators, empowering our clients to learn skills to change and evolve.

One of the skills needed to successfully ride the waves of life's changes is flexibility. If your clients are not flexible in challenging their perceptions and their old ways of doing things, they will continue to play worn-out life themes.

Clients who seek help in counseling but are not able to shift their perceptions and change their ways of coping typically become treatment resistant and often do not last long in therapy. The healthier that individuals are, the more likely it is that they possess mental and emotional flexibility.

Jan was a nurse manager who claimed she "hated" change. Of course, her job in the hospital involved a constant state of change, and she found that she was less and less able to keep up with the demands of her job and to juggle her responsibilities at home with a husband and two young children. She came to counseling after having a meltdown when her husband invited his stepsiblings for Thanksgiving, which would increase the number at the table from 12 to 14. Jan was angry at him for not consulting with her first and upset that she had enough place settings for only 12 people. Her resistance to change was based on a need to have things "perfect." She was not sure if she could set a nice table for 14, and felt as if things had spiraled out of control. The work I did with Jan ended up focusing on her perfectionism, rigidity, and strong need to control most aspects of her life. Jan learned that, in order to enjoy life more, she needed to give up her need to control and have everything "just so." She realized that her rigidity and need to have things perfect were causing her to be stressed with her daughters. With Jan, I used traditional Cognitive Behavior Therapy (CBT) techniques, such as helping her identify her rigid, irrational thoughts and replacing those thoughts with more flexible and healthier ones. For example, she learned to replace her catastrophic "It's *terrible!*" with milder terms such as "It's annoying" or "It's disappointing." By limiting her cognitive distortions, Jan began to learn to be more flexible with unexpected life changes. I used other flexibility exercises with Jan as outlined in the following treatment tips section.

Treatment Tips

☑ ACT Technique: Cognitive Defusion

On his website, Acceptance and Commitment Therapy (ACT) founder Steven Hayes, offers various techniques to help clients use cognitive defusion to cope with distress and basically become less "fused" with unhealthy ways of thinking by developing more of a non-judgmental, objective view of their upsetting thoughts. Here are a few examples to use as a springboard to help clients change.

- Instead of thinking "I'm a loser," clients can be taught to distance themselves from that thought and replace it thought with the more objective "I am having the thought that I am a loser."
- Instead of believing the thought that "I will never change," clients can be taught to objectively evaluate what type of cognitive distortion that thought results from, such as "There I go again, fortune telling!"
- Help clients learn to "just notice" things instead of evaluating and interpreting situations with a judgmental stance.
- Have clients sound out their difficult thoughts by saying them slowly out loud—instead of having them on unquestioned autopilot.
- Have clients lighten up about their irrational and upsetting thoughts by saying the thoughts as different characters, such as Donald Duck. This helps keep them in perspective.
- Have clients sing out the upsetting thoughts—again, to lighten up about them and distance themselves from the intensity of emotions.

☑ Exercise: Get a Grip!

This simple—yet very effective—exercise has been a great tool for my therapeutic toolbox. In individual as well as group sessions, this exercise helps clients appreciate the importance of flexibility in adapting to change and illustrates the importance of shifting perceptions and being open-minded instead of maintaining rigid ways of thinking.

I begin by asking my clients to clasp their hands with their fingers interlocked. I then ask, "Which thumb is on top?" In a group situation, about half will have their left thumb on top and half will have the right on top, regardless of whether they are right or left-handed. What is natural for some is not natural for another. I make the point that this represents our perceptions—we think people see things the same way, and this exercise proves that this is not true.

I then ask my clients to shift their fingers so that the other thumb is on top, with the rest of the fingers following suit. I ask them, "How does it feel?" Common responses are "weird," "strange," and "uncomfortable." However, for some people it is effortless and natural! Thus, this exercise serves as a demonstration of how we need to shift our thinking just slightly in order to see things in a different way and adapt to life's changing demands.

For even more impact, I ask my clients to fold their arms, noticing which arm is on top and then to switch so that the other arm is on top. Some people keep rolling their arms, unable to find a comfortable position. Between the laughter and smiles, the point is well made that only by being flexible can we change our perceptions and look at things from other points of view. The way we do things is not the only right way!

In my sessions, I sometimes intertwine my fingers or fold my arms (just like in the exercise) to show my clients that they are digging themselves into holes with their rigid, inflexible thinking. That gesture has become a running joke between some clients and me over the years, and they show me their fingers interlocked or arms folded when they recognize that they are falling into a rigid way of thinking. This visual becomes a call to action to shift perceptions.

☑ Activity: Changing Places

Another short and simple exercise I like to do with my clients is to have them switch seats. With individual clients, I have them switch seats with me, or just sit in a different chair in my office. In groups, I have participants switch places with one another and briefly talk about their reaction to the exercise. We then discuss how it feels to change and talk about some of the benefits and drawbacks of the new seat. This exercise helps them experience emotions related to change. In individual situations, clients often claim they see the room from a different view and notice things they hadn't noticed before. In a group situation, they often say they get a chance to sit next to different people. If the group seems happy to change seats, have them do it another time or two to get a chance to connect with different people, asking them a question or giving them a topic to discuss each time. This is a nice team-building exercise.

☑ *Activity: Changing Appearances*

A very popular group exercise is one in which clients change things about their physical appearance. This exercise emphasizes that change can be fun and not something that should be resisted. Pair off into partners and have them stand facing away from each other, and then have them make some changes, such as removing a watch, unbuttoning extra buttons, or taking off glasses. Then have them face each other and describe the changes that the other person made.

To make this into a bit of a game, play another round by pairing up the winners (those who guessed more items correctly than their partner in the previous round) while the others watch. Play as many rounds as necessary until only the most observant and mindful person in the group is still standing. These additional winners rounds reinforce to group members that those who are mindful and observant through life—rather than those with tunnel vision—will be more likely to be "winners" in life.

☑ *Activity: Switching Sides*

Another quick and fun group activity is to have everyone switch their watches, bracelets, scarves, and other clothing accessories from one side to the other. Have them process how it feels. Suggest that they try putting their watch or bracelet on the opposite arm for the next week, and then discuss at the next session how it felt to make these changes and what they can learn from this exercise about "switching sides."

☑ *Activity: Riddles and Brainteasers*

In group situations, brainteasers are a fun way to help clients change their thinking and look at things in a new and creative way. The brainteasers below are representative of puzzling life situations and emphasize the importance of thinking creatively. They can be shown either on a handout or on a PowerPoint presentation.

Ask your clients what the word or phrase each puzzle represents.

Riddles are another way that I teach flexible and creative problem solving in groups. For example, when I ask, "What is the largest room in the world?" I get responses such as "the Taj Majal" or "Versailles," but in actuality, the largest room in the world is *the room for improvement*! A fun

---

BRAINTEASERS

1. BACK	2. BENDING	3. HISTORY	4. _____
BA	_____	HISTORY	READ
B __	__KCAB	HISTORY	_____

5. **BIRD** 6. O-ER-T-O- 7. RcAaErG 8. SIRDKN
                                             ISRKND
                                           DNRKSI

ANSWER: 1. Full Back, Half Back, Quarterback 2. Bending over backwards 3. History repeats itself 4. Reading between the lines 5. BigBird 6. Painless Operation 7. Car in reverse gear 8. Mixed Drinks

group activity, even with children and teens, is to share riddles, making the point that all riddles require flexible thinking to "get it."

☑ Exercise: Equation Puzzle

This puzzle is another brainteaser that illustrates the importance of flexible thinking. You can use this example with individuals, but I usually use it in a group situation.

I ask group members if they would rather have a million dollars or a penny that doubles every day of a 30-day month. Most participants will take the penny, assuming that their choice results in more money. However, once I start upping the ante and asking for volunteers to take $2 million, and then $3 million, and then $4 million, there are many who offer to take the money and run. So what's the difference between the two choices? $1,000,000 vs. $5,386,709.12!

☑ Metaphors and Analogies: Creative ways Facilitate Change

As therapists, we can help our clients develop more mental flexibility by using metaphors and exercises to help them expand their perceptions and open their minds. As I have mentioned, the third-wave treatment modalities such as ACT, DBT, and MBCT utilize creative practices that make use of acronyms, metaphors, and visualizations. CBT also uses such practices, but the third-wave approach relies on them as a cornerstone of treatment.

The third-wave approaches (especially ACT) focus on flexibility as a core concept of the entire model. ACT bases its theory on a model of six core psychopathological processes (such as avoidance and lack of values clarity), and the hub of these processes is called *psychological inflexibility*. This is precisely why ACT is rich in experiential exercises and the use of metaphors and visualizations which elicit flexibility.

There are a number of ways that we can help liberate our clients from change paralysis. The only thing that limits us is our own imagination. At times, I have felt like a cult deprogrammer when helping people depart from their rigid ways of thinking. And many times their problem stems from a history of dominating parents and/or some type of abuse. Clients who have learned shame-based ways of thinking have invisible loyalties to a rigid sense of what is right and what is wrong, and they lack trust in themselves to shift their perceptions and look at things in new ways, not knowing if they would be "right."

In these cases, changing their way of thinking becomes almost like a betrayal—for example, disloyalty to the parents they love, despite the parents' aggressive and dominating personalities. In cases like this, metaphors and visualizations are especially powerful in tackling emotionally crippling change resistance. Jeannie, a 34-year old nurse, came for counseling to address her debilitating anxiety and fear of her domineering boss. She feared receiving snide comments or any type of perceived criticism and constantly felt on edge because she thought her boss was talking behind her back. It didn't take her long to discover that her manager reminded her of her judgmental and disapproving father. Even though she was well into her 30s and had a family of her own, she felt compelled to get her father's approval for common life decisions, such as where to go to church and what car to buy. If she didn't get his approval, she felt even more anxious, like she was doing something "bad" or, even worse, that she was bad herself. She confided, "I feel guilty all the time, even if I'm not doing anything wrong." She also felt guilty even mentioning anything about her father, and felt like she was betraying him by talking behind his back.

For Jeannie, it was a big step to come to counseling and share with me about the situation with her father. I needed to handle what she told me gingerly, as it is not uncommon for clients to drop out of therapy if they feel guilty about betraying a loved one. I reassured her that a counselor's office is where you can process things without feeling as if you are betraying confidence or "invisible loyalties," and that she was not "wrong" or "bad." I also reassured her that it was clear that she loved her father and that her father loved her, but that it was likely that he had not treated her in a healthy way when she was a child because he just didn't know any better. The reassurance that unhealthy people are not bad people, and that part of her father's unhealthiness was that he didn't know he was unhealthy, was a comfort to her. After all, we were working on helping her, not condemning him. My analogy of needing to learn a new, healthier language (as mentioned in Chapter 8) was quite helpful to her. She had never before realized that the shame-based, faulty language she had learned was not a correct one, because that was the only language her family knew. She became excited about the opportunity to learn to "translate" that language into one that would give her a more positive life, and one that she could teach her children.

This, I helped Jeannie break out of her shame-based thinking using the analogy of learning a new language. I have found this analogy very useful in helping clients to unlock their change paralysis. In Jeannie's case, this new perspective released her from her alliance to her unhealthy interpretations and removed old habits of coping that did not work well in her life and caused excessive approval-seeking behavior. Her mood and anxiety started to lift, and her confidence rose.

I also found it helpful with Jeannie, as with many other clients, to unleash the power of other analogies and metaphors. The following are some other metaphors and analogies that can be used to unlock change paralysis.

METAPHORS: TRANSFORMATIONS ARE A BEAUTIFUL PART OF NATURE
One of my favorite metaphors of change and transformation is captured in the image of a caterpillar, incubating in a cocoon, and emerging as a beautiful, colorful butterfly. The old proverb "Just when the caterpillar

thought the world was over, it became a butterfly" is one I remind my clients of when they need faith and hope that they can get through difficult changes in their lives. As they grow and change through therapy, they can emerge like butterflies and their souls can take wing and soar. The sunflower is another of my favorite metaphors; if clients seek positivity as the sunflower seeks light, they will grow tall and beautiful.

ACT METAPHORS: UNLOCKING INFLEXIBILITY

The Big Book of ACT Metaphors (Stoddard & Afari, 2014) offers many metaphors from various ACT therapists that can be used in unlocking psychological inflexibility.

One of the sections of the book, *Taking Off Your Armor* uses the metaphor of armor to symbolize how individuals protect themselves from hurt due to past trauma, as well as from change. The armor becomes a way of life, even when the protection is no longer needed. Using this image, you can ask clients if they still need such protection now that their life has changed, or if it is preventing them from growing. By inviting your client to remove the armor, you can invite them to love themselves and others more freely.

One popular ACT metaphor that I use often is a beach ball. Resisting change or resisting your thoughts instead of making peace with them is like trying to push an inflated beach ball under the water—it keeps on popping up! In helping your clients to stop resisting change, you can use this metaphor to illustrate a futile task. You might even want to use a tub of water and a beach ball to demonstrate how hard it is to resist change. These demonstrations make a great impact—and make a big splash!

Another popular ACT metaphor, which was developed by ACT founder Steven Hayes, is called "passengers on the bus." In this visualization, Hayes suggests seeing yourself driving a bus. Each passenger represents critical, judgmental thoughts being shouted at you. Imagine yourself not reacting, but keeping focused on the road ahead, guided by your own values and direction. This metaphor can help clients achieve a sense of mastery over their thoughts. Through the imagery described, clients experience the confidence to drive their own destiny and not allow critical voices to sidetrack them.

MINI-LESSON: DANGER PLUS OPPORTUNITY

An interesting image that was actually referred to by President John F. Kennedy represents the resilience to change that adversity offers us. The image that JFK referred to—which I commonly use in my seminars and groups—is that of the Chinese symbol for *crisis*. It is made up of two symbols, or words, representing *danger* plus *opportunity*. This is a great example of how even unsought and threatening changes offer opportunities for us, as long as we open new doors once some other door has closed.

CRISIS

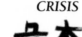

Danger *plus* Opportunity

☑ *Activity: Quick Quizzes to Facilitate Flexibility and Change*

HUMOR INVENTORY

This chapter would not be complete without mentioning the importance of humor in facilitating growth and change. After all, a sense of humor is no laughing matter. It's important stuff! You don't have to be funny to have a sense of humor—rather, it is an attitude that sees the "bright side of life," as Monty Python would say. It's a tool to use to handle life's everyday up and downs—and changes. It's a coping strategy for flowing and adapting to the unpredictability of life. This quick "Humor Inventory" (Handout 10.4) was developed to help clients get in the mindset to remember to use their sense of humor, and to get a quick gauge of their Humor Quotient. This worksheet is great for individual clients and groups, stressing the importance of using humor in everyday life. You can use this periodically with a client to see if their Humor Quotient improves, particularly for those who scored low previously.

WELLNESS INVENTORY

"How Is Your 'Mental Wellness'?" (Handout 10.5) offers a quick gauge of emotional and mental wellness via a short, eight-item quiz. In this inventory, questions are geared toward covering the general areas of mental wellness, such as feeling satisfied with oneself and others, not holding grudges, handling change optimistically, feeling in control over one's life, and having a sense of gratitude. If your clients score low, consider having them fill this out periodically to see if they are able to boost their mental wellness IQ.

☑ Activity: Tracking Change Resiliency

As in all the other chapters, remember to offer your clients daily logs and weekly summary logs to help them work on their therapeutic goals. In relation to change resiliency, the "Reaction to Life Changes Log" (Handouts 10.2 and 10.3) as well as the "Weekly Change Log" (Handout 10.6) offer your clients a way to track their progress.

☑ Activity: Thinking Back: The Pros and Cons

When change resistance and fear of the future and of the unknown make it difficult for clients to progress in therapy, I ask them to imagine one of the most challenging and difficult times they've ever experienced. Together, we then list the pros and cons of coping with this adversity, describing how it has strengthened them and how it has weakened them. You can make a list like this in the session with your client:

Example of Personal Adversity

How I Became Weaker	*How I Became Deeper*

Even if they wish the adversity had not occurred, I ask them to think about how that deepening, change, and growth has helped them become part of who they are today. I also question whether they would want to trade that depth of character if they could. This exercise helps clients see that even difficult change has its advantages, and it is up to them to decide how they'll respond to it in order to deepen rather than weaken.

☑ Activity: Manage Change While Having a Ball!

Change is a great topic for group activities, and who can't relate to the importance of being flexible? The group activity below is a fun and engaging stress-filled exercise that helps clients experience the sweetness and fun of change, and learn how to master it. This activity is bound to get a lot of laughs and smiles while making the point of how sweet change really is!

This short yet powerful group activity utilizes stress balls to highlight key points about change resiliency and encourages active group engagement. The main purpose of this activity is to illustrate that change can be stressful, but it can also be fun—even if you drop the ball and make mistakes along the way!

ACTIVITY STRUCTURE

1. Participants form circles of anywhere from five to eight people.
2. Give one person in each circle a foam stress ball with the instruction that he or she is not to throw it to someone, but not someone who is standing right next to him or her. The receiver of the ball then throws it to someone else who didn't have a turn yet, until everyone has had a turn and the ball is back with the original person.
3. Have the group members throw the ball again, repeating the same pattern a couple of times in the same exact order until they have memorized the pattern.
4. Once they have perfected the pattern, have them go a bit faster, a few more times.
5. Then introduce another ball, and then another and then

another. Thus, it goes from one ball, to two, to three, to four, and so forth, until the number of balls equals the number of people in the group.

6. Have more stress balls ready so the participants don't have to chase down dropped balls. Keep supplying balls so that the number of balls equals the number of people in the group.

7. Keep up the activity for just a couple minutes, and expect a lot of laughter and surprise as the new balls are introduced.

8. After having people take their seats, ask them how this exercise helps to represent stress and how to manage it. What did they learn about managing change and being flexible to adjust to all those new balls and demands made on them?

HERE ARE SOME KEY POINTS FOR THE DISCUSSION:

Change and flexibility can be fun! Make the point that this activity is proof that stress can be fun and positive.

Stay focused and directed. In order to keep the exercise going, participants can't get distracted by what other people are doing. Rather, the ability to master the demands of each new ball comes from focusing on where the ball comes from and where it is going. Being focused on your goal is the key to success.

It's okay to make mistakes. The more the balls were dropped, the more laughter there was—demonstrating that mistakes are not horrible and, in fact, made the activity more fun.

To enjoy the activity, we need to be flexible. At the start of the activity, no one has a clue that more than one ball will be introduced. Once they are, group members adapt quite quickly and seem pleasantly surprised at the new twist in the activity.

Being mindful and focused on the present can help manage adapting to change. During this activity, everyone is mentally present and focused, proving that staying in the present helps productivity. Instead of thinking about what they're having for dinner that night or what happened yesterday, participants remained focused in the present. Make the point that a non-judgmental focus helps them adapt to change. If we focus too much on the past or future, we will get bombarded with the balls. This is a great activity for teaching the concept of mindfulness.

☑ Activity: Mindful Awareness

Another quick and easy exercise for helping clients to become centered in the present and develop mindful awareness is to have group participants look around them and find all the things that are of a certain color, like black.

After they close their eyes, ask them to name all the things that they observed in green! This exercise drives home the point that when we are looking for some things in our environment, we are not observant about other things, and thus our perceptions are skewed toward what we are looking for. This reveals how we see others and ourselves. If we are looking for the selfishness or the "bad" in a person, we will find much to criticize. If we look for the good, we will also find it.

To quote Author Anais Nin, "We don't see things as they are, we see them as we are."

☑ Mini-Lesson: Learning the Stages of Change

Even though most clients come voluntarily for counseling, they might not be ready to commit themselves to major changes. Sometimes they come to get help in certain areas and may not be receptive to working on other areas.

Linda and Doug came to me office for marriage counseling. Doug's stated purpose of coming was to get Linda to see how cold she was, and he wanted more affection. Linda wanted him to stop drinking excessively so she could feel warmer toward him. When the topic of Doug's excessive drinking came up, he became defensive and denied it was a problem. Linda ended up going to counseling alone after that first session, as Doug told her that if she brought his drinking up, he was "out of there." Thus, he was ready for her to fix her problems, but he was not ready to make a change himself.

This example illustrates the importance of evaluating a client's "readiness for change." This is a focus of Motivational Interviewing, originated in 1983 by psychologists William Miller and Stephen Rollnick. Miller found that clients who abused alcohol often became resistant in counseling when the focus became too centered around the alcohol use. The key to motivational interviewing (developed further by Prochaska and DiClemente's stages of change model [Prochaska, Norcross, & DiClemente, 1994]) is the client's readiness to change, and consideration of this is essential in solution-oriented therapy.

For instance, if a client is not ready for solutions and is still ambivalent about needing to change, patience and active listening are essential therapeutic skills to use until there is more readiness and less denial. Some clients who come to counseling may not be ready for life-altering skill building if they don't have the insight that they need to change. They still might think their problems are because of someone else. It is not uncommon to see a client in therapy who thinks that it is their spouse, boss, or parents who are at the root of their problem, and that if only *they* would change, life would be so much better.

All too often, therapists do not sufficiently evaluate or consider where the client is on the readiness-to-change continuum. Even if clients come to counseling on their own because of some major life event, this doesn't mean they are emotionally ready to change their ingrained habits. If a client is ambivalent about the need to change, they are in the precontemplation stage of change, the first stage.

Following are the five stages of change; where clients are on this continuum determines their degree of readiness. If therapists are not sensitive to their stage of readiness, clients may be lost unnecessarily through dropping out of treatment. Only when therapeutic efforts are in sync with the client's level of readiness can the real healing begin.

THE FIVE STAGES OF CHANGE

> **Precontemplation.** Clients are using avoidance and are not ready to change. An example could be a wife coming in for treatment not thinking that she herself has a problem, or vice versa (a husband not thinking he has a problem).

Contemplation. Clients are ambivalent about wanting to change and give up long-standing habits. They are still weighing the pros and cons of change and evaluating the discrepancies between their behavior and goals.

Preparation/determination. Clients are taking steps to change.

Action/willpower. Clients are using new behaviors and learning new skills and habits.

Maintenance. Clients have integrated healthy changes in behavior into their life.

A Toolkit of Metaphors for Change Resistance

The following are some metaphorical items representing change resistance. A fun group activity is to have clients make up a metaphorical toolkit to embrace change.

A coin. I often have participants look for change in their pockets to represent that change is all around us—even in our back pocket!

A kaleidoscope. I have gotten these online and given them out to workshop participants to remind them that change can be beautiful in its colorfulness and unpredictability.

A pencil. You can rewrite your life story, and the changes you make are under your control.

A popcorn packet. Put the popcorn in a microwave, and it is transformed in 4 minutes or less. How's that for positive change?

A snow globe. Shake it and everything changes!

A picture of a butterfly. Life involves transformations, and change can bring about something very beautiful.

Can you and your client think of others?

Therapeutic Takeaways

☑ Change is good—we all need change to evolve, grow, and thrive. We become resistant to change when we feel it is out of our control.

☑ Change requires flexibility, and exercises and activities that help clients become more flexible in their thinking will help limit their change resistance.

☑ The use of metaphors unlocks change resistance.

☑ Psychoeducation can help clients learn to deepen instead of weaken in the face of life change.

☑ Solution-oriented therapists are like language teachers and translators, teaching their clients a new emotional language.

☑ Solution-oriented therapists need to be mindful of the stages of change and make sure they are attentive to where each client fits on the continuum.

Handouts

The following worksheets will help your clients build their change-resistance skills. These worksheets are all related to the lessons of this chapter. As a general guideline, handouts and assignments are given to clients at the end of the session as homework, unless they are used in the session itself to illustrate points. Make sure you leave ample time to go over your expectations regarding your clients' use of the selected handouts.

When assignments are given out, it is important to follow up with your clients at the beginning of the next session by reviewing and discussing their homework with them. Going over homework is an essential aspect of being a solution-oriented therapist.

Note: All handouts in the book are available for download on my website by following the link below: http://www.belmontwellness.com/ultimate-solution-handouts/

Handout 10.1: Common Myths About Change

Myth 1: The most important changes come from the outside.

Although change is all around us, some of the most important changes we can make in our lives involve our own perceptions. To quote Wayne Dyer, "If you change the way you look at things, the things you look at change." Most of us underestimate the power of attitude and the importance of changing the way we look at things. Happiness does not come mostly from outside of us. All too often, getting a nicer car, a newer and bigger house, or talented children does not give us the happiness we seek. Happiness is an inside job.

Myth 2: People need to change for us to be happier with ourselves and them.

Some people spend their lives looking to change things around them—including other people—when they really need to be focused on changing themselves and how they cope. It is okay to ask others for a change, but too often people put their happiness and well-being on hold as they wait for others to change. The problem is that we end up becoming aggressive if we try to change someone else, when really the only person we can change is ourselves.

Myth 3: Change is avoidable.

Whether we like it or not, things never stay the same. Life is in a constant state of evolution, and trying to keep things as they are will make you emotionally stagnant. Avoiding change is like fighting against the ocean tides—it is so much easier to flow with the tides of change, adapt to them, and be flexible than it is to try to alter the forces of nature.

Myth 4: Change is often a reaction to outside forces.

To the contrary, meaningful change comes more from our own self-motivation than from motivation from outside forces. People often resist change because they don't like to feel like they are *being* changed. But if we are involved in our changes and they are not imposed on us—whether they be personal or workplace change—we are more likely to adapt.

For those in a position of leadership, it is important to keep in mind people's need to be part of the change they are going through rather than having it imposed on them. A sense of control is a key factor in overcoming change resistance.

Handout 10.2: Reaction to Life Changes Log

With Handout 10.3 serving as a model, use this log to help you more effectively cope with life changes.

Current Situation	
Negative Emotions	Positive Emotions
Strength of Negative Emotions 1 2 3 4 5 6 7 8 9 10 Low High	Strength of Positive Emotions 1 2 3 4 5 6 7 8 9 10 Low High
Identify Negative Beliefs	Challenge With Positive Beliefs
Type of Cognitive Error	Response to Cognitive Error
Certainty of Your Beliefs 1 2 3 4 5 6 7 8 9 10 Low High	Certainty of Your Beliefs 1 2 3 4 5 6 7 8 9 10 Low High
Unhealthy Reactions to Change	Healthy Reactions to Change
Cost/Benefit Analysis: Unhealthy Coping With Change	Cost/Benefit Analysis: Healthy Coping With Change
My Conclusions and Goals	

Handout 10.3: Reaction to Life Changes Log, Completed

Current Situation	
Difficulty adjusting to new job right after graduation from college	
Negative Emotions	**Positive Emotions**
Afraid, intimidated	Excited, hopeful
Strength of Negative Emotions	**Strength of Positive Emotions**
_____X_____ 1 2 3 4 5 6 7 8 9 10 Low High	_____X_____ 1 2 3 4 5 6 7 8 9 10 Low High
Identify Negative Beliefs	**Challenge With Positive Beliefs**
They might regret hiring me - I'm not smart like a lot of the others. It would be TERRIBLE to make a mistake	I need to stop comparing myself with others. They know I have little experience and just graduated. It's OK to make mistakes.
Type of Cognitive Error	**Response to Cognitive Error**
Over-catastrophizing, all or nothing thinking, making comparisons	I will stick to the facts. I will only compare myself to myself before today - not others
Certainty of Your Beliefs	**Certainty of Your Beliefs**
_____X_____ 1 2 3 4 5 6 7 8 9 10 Low High	_____X____ 1 2 3 4 5 6 7 8 9 10 Low High
Unhealthy Reactions to Change	**Healthy Reactions to Change**
Withdraw after work, isolate myself	Will try to make new friends at work, ask them to lunch for example
Cost/Benefit Analysis: **Unhealthy Coping With Change**	**Cost/Benefit Analysis:** **Healthy Coping With Change**
Will feel stressed and depressed	Will meet new people and be open to new experiences
My Conclusions and Goals	
I will get nothing out of isolating and being intimidated. I will use this new job as a chance to embrace change and grow from it professionally and personally.	

Handout 10.4: Humor Inventory

Life is too serious to be taken so seriously! Laughter, smiles, and positive thinking all are ingredients of a sense of humor. A sense of humor will help you to see the bright side of life and to be resilient in meeting the challenges of everyday life. Sometimes we get so caught up in problems that we do not see the solutions.

The following questions will help you take stock of your "humor inventory."

Rate each item on the following scale:

False _____ True

| 1 | 2 | 3 | 4 | 5 |

_____ 1. I have a hard time seeing the humor in everyday life.

_____ 2. I am usually too stressed and busy to enjoy the moment.

_____ 3. I get so caught up in my stresses that I rarely look at the lighter side of life.

_____ 4. I find myself holding too many grudges, resentments, and bitterness.

_____ 5. In general, I rarely find things to laugh about, and I know I take myself too seriously.

_____ 6. I have a hard time adapting to change, and generally like things to stay the same.

_____ 7. I have not had a good laugh in quite some time and do not smile enough.

Take your total score and divide it by 7:

Total score _____ divided by 7 equals your score: _____ .

Interpretation of Your Score

1 Superb: Your Humor Quotient is unusually high! Keep up the good work!
2 Very Good: Your lightness of attitude helps you to be stress-hardy.
3 Average: Your Humor Quotient is average and could use some boosting.
4 Needs Work: Look for more opportunities to lighten up.
5 You are more prone to emotional and physical problems: Life is too serious to be taken so seriously! Consider getting professional help.

Handout 10.5: How Is Your "Mental Wellness?"

Emotional and mental wellness is a determinant of life satisfaction, physical health, and even how long you live. We all know the importance of physical fitness, but being mentally and emotionally fit is equally important. The following quiz will give you a snapshot of your "mental wellness IQ"

Below are eight items to rate your degree of agreement. On a scale of 1 to 7, rate how much you agree with each item. These items represent some of the major factors in mental wellness.

1	2	3	4	5	6	7
Strongly disagree		Neither Agree nor Disagree			Strongly Agree	

_____ 1. I feel satisfied with who I am and where I am in my life.

_____ 2. I refuse to allow regrets and disappointments to cloud "today."

_____ 3. I feel a strong sense of connection with others and do not feel isolated.

_____ 4. I tend to think rationally and optimistically, even in times of life changes.

_____ 5. I can forgive others for not living up to my expectations and have no grudges.

_____ 6. I feel a great sense of control over my emotions, thoughts, and feelings.

_____ 7. I have a healthy sense of humor and laugh at life's imperfections—and my own.

_____ 8. I focus more on being grateful for how my life is now than on what's lacking in my life.

51–56 You have the highest degree of mental wellness. Congratulations!

46–50 Your mental wellness is very high, and you have a very good attitude.

40–46 Your mental wellness is moderate and is a cause for concern. Caution!

32–39 Your mental wellness is borderline. Work on changing your attitude.

24–31 Your lack of mental well-being is likely going to interfere with your physical and mental health.

16–23 You are heading into a danger zone. Get professional help and invest time in improving your attitude.

Below 15 Danger zone! You need professional help immediately to avoid severe depression.

Handout 10.6: Weekly Change Log

Date(s): _____

1. Example of changing event (s):

_____

2. My emotional responses:

_____

3. Degree of negative reaction to stress:

                        LOW 1 2 3 4 5 6 7 8 9 10 HIGH

4. Unhealthy thoughts:

_____

    Certainty of beliefs: LOW 1 2 3 4 5 6 7 8 9 10 HIGH

5. Types of cognitive distortions:

_____

6. Healthy thoughts:

_____

    Certainty of beliefs: LOW 1 2 3 4 5 6 7 8 9 10 HIGH

7. Unhealthy reactions to change:

_____

8. Healthy reactions to change:

_____

9. Mindfulness and acceptance skills I have practiced:

_____

10. Metaphors and visualizations I have used:

_____

11. Alternative skills I can use to cope with change:

_____

12. Costs and benefits of my healthy and unhealthy thinking:

_____

13. Goals for managing change and improving my coping skills:

_____

Recommended Resources

Self-Help Books

The Swiss Cheese Theory of Life: How to Get Through Life's Holes Without Getting Stuck in Them!
Judith A. Belmont and Lora Shor

Feeling Good: The New Mood Therapy
David D. Burns

Change Your Thoughts, Change Your Life: Living the Wisdom of the Tao
Wayne W. Dyer

Who Moved My Cheese? An A-Mazing Way to Deal With Change in Your Work and in Your Life
Spencer Johnson

Clinician Books

Motivational Interviewing: Helping People Change
William R. Miller and Stephen Rollnick

Changing for Good: A Revolutionary Six-Stage Program for Overcoming Bad Habits and Moving Your Life Positively Forward
James O. Prochaska, John C. Norcross, and Carlo C. DiClemente

The Big Book of ACT Metaphors: A Practitioner's Guide to Experiential Exercises & Metaphors in Acceptance & Commitment Therapy
Jill A. Stoddard and Niloofar Afari

Links

Association for Contextual Behavioral Science
"Cognitive Defusion Strategies (Delateralization)" by Steven Hayes
http://contextualscience.org/cognitive_defusion_deliteralization

Worksheets and handouts from ACT's Russ Harris
http://www.actmindfully.com.au

Motivational Interviewing
http://www.motivationalinterview.org

Stephen Rollnick
http://www.stephenrollnick.com

CHAPTER ELEVEN

Putting Solutions Into Practice
10 Ultimate Therapeutic Solutions

As you can see in this *Ultimate Solution Book*, there are certain universal characteristics of solution-oriented treatment for any client problem. This last chapter will offer a summary of 10 important solution-oriented strategies to incorporate into your toolkit that will offer your client skills for a lifetime.

You have seen these 10 universal strategies throughout the book time and time again, individualized and tailored to specific client issues. At the end of this chapter, there will be a checklist for you to use as you devise your own solution-oriented treatment approach.

☑ 1. Use Psychoeducation to Teach Clients in Almost Every Session

The role of the therapist is to listen, to talk, *and to teach*. Offering clients an array of worksheets, logs, handouts, visualizations, activities, and mini-lessons will provide them with self-help skills to last a lifetime. Make sure you have in your office plenty of handouts to offer clients based on the skills they need to work on. It may also be beneficial to provide folders, which will help your clients keep their handouts organized as they bring them back and forth between sessions.

It is important to note that psychoeducation is not meant to *tell* clients what to do, but rather to *educate* clients so that they can develop the skills they need to find solutions to their problems.

☑ 2. Start Each Session With a Mood Check

Starting off the session with a question like "How did you feel this past week?" is an example of an informal mood check. It's usually brief and provides an idea of how the client is doing.

More formal mood checks include the Beck Depression Inventory and the Burns Depression Inventory. These are particularly important for high-risk and suicidal clients (or severely depressed clients). Having your clients take these inventories frequently, even in some cases at each session, will help you to identify severe depression that might require further intervention, such as hospitalization or more frequent sessions. The resources for these mood and depression inventories are included in the resources section at the end of Chapter 3, and inventories for other symptoms, such as the Burns Anxiety Inventory, are included in the relevant chapters. For your convenience, I have included in the link section at the end of this chapter the website links of some of the most influential psychoeducational practitioners mentioned frequently in this book, which offer their most widely used inventories, quick tests, and mood check forms.

This brief part of the session can also include, if appropriate, a medication check, in which you ask clients whether they have any reactions or medication-related issues they would like to discuss.

☑ 3. Start Each Session by Clarifying Goals

The beginning part of the session is also a time to clarify goals for the session. Asking your client questions such as "Do you have any goals for today? " or "What would you like to work on today?" will help ensure that you are addressing your client's needs and goals and not getting sidetracked by your own agenda.

In Cognitive Behavior Therapy (CBT), Judith Beck emphasizes that successful treatment is goal oriented and problem focused. Goal setting at the beginning of every session is important and starts the session off on a collaborative note (J. S. Beck, 2011).

At times, the goals of client and therapist may clash, and letting the client set the agenda and goals (often with the therapist's input, of course) will help lessen the possibility of resistance. For example, if you think the client's real issue is his denial of his alcohol problem, but he wants to focus on his relationship with his spouse, the client will be much less resistant and more engaged if his agenda—not yours—is the focus for the session. There certainly can be mention of how alcohol use might be a source of strain in the relationship, but that doesn't mean the focus of the session should be breaking through the denial. In fact, trying to break through the denial before the client is ready is a surefire way to undermine therapy or even lose a client. This is why learning about Motivational Interviewing is so crucial; it emphasizes the importance of evaluating the client's stage of readiness to change in formulating a treatment plan. In Motivational Interviewing, the increasingly popular goal-directed counseling approach developed by Rollnick and Miller, evaluating clients' readiness to change ensures that the therapist is nonjudgmental and doesn't push clients to develop insights or to make changes they are not yet willing to make (such as stopping addictive behaviors).

In Dialectical Behavior Therapy (DBT), Marsha Linehan also emphasizes the importance of goal setting. She identifies setting concrete goals and behavioral targets as crucial to therapeutic success—with the overall goal being "having a life worth living." In DBT, therapists who are validating will focus on goal setting with their clients at the start of a session (Linehan, 1993).

Thus, making it a habit to ask your client "What is your goal for today?" at the beginning of the session is a simple way of putting their goals into focus, and can be just what is needed to make the session an effective, solution-oriented one.

☑ 4. Use Creative Visualizations and Experiential Activities

Confucius is quoted to have said, "Tell me, and I will forget. Show me and I may remember. Involve me, and I will understand." I often use this exact quote to start off my PowerPoint presentations for my professional seminars as well as my workplace wellness presentations.

This quote epitomizes a crucial ingredient of any solution-oriented therapy—engaging a client with visualizations and experiential activities to make learning come alive. This is why, in solution-oriented therapy, individual and group clients often *do* rather than just *talk*. Whether it is role playing, filling out handouts, filling out diaries and logs, or engaging in experiential group activities to illustrate a psychoeducational lesson, clients are engaged in practicing new skills.

The use of visualizations in treatment follows the adage "A picture is worth a thousand words." Visualization can help clients understand concepts and accept them when words alone cannot reach them. Therapist-guided visualizations are quite powerful, as clients are led to use their imaginations and be mindful of their thoughts and sensations in the process of healing.

An especially effective visualization, explained in Chapter 3, is one used frequently in Mindfulness-Based Cognitive Therapy (MBCT) and Acceptance and Commitment Therapy (ACT): "Leaves floating on a stream." Imagining that each leaf has a worrisome or disturbing thought, and watching these thoughts float out of your head and down the stream in many different directions until they disappear, will help your clients become more rational and objective about their disturbing thoughts.

Guided progressive relaxation, such as the MBCT body scan, helps clients learn systematic ways to relax by focusing on various parts of the body while breathing deeply and relaxing certain body muscles.

These above examples are just a sample of the vast array of visualizations that clinicians use to help clients heal.

☑ 5. Use Self-Help Assignments Between Sessions

Perhaps one of the most important aspects of CBT and *third-wave* cognitive therapies is an emphasis on *self-help assignments*. Although it is often referred to as *homework*, I prefer the term *self-help assignments*, since the word *homework* is less empowering and can have some deep-seated associations with memories of difficult school experiences, and has the connotation of being imposed from the outside. The term *self-help assignments* affirms the need for clients to be proactive rather than passive in their learning. CBT clinicians also use terms like *practice*, *experiments* and *action plan* to refer to between-session assignments.

An analogy made in the Introduction that deserves to be repeated is that of a music student learning a musical instrument. Lessons are only an opportunity to learn new skills, but practice during the week will be what the student needs in order to progress. Therapy is much like this. If an individual comes to sessions but does not work between sessions, progress will be significantly handicapped.

Self-help assignments are tailored to individual treatment needs. If a client is anxious, exposure techniques in which the client faces his or her fear would be an example of working between sessions. Filling out worksheets to learn to challenge irrational thoughts and reading a self-help book or reviewing handouts are some other examples of ways to help an anxious client learn ways to lessen their anxiety. Practicing assertive skills in front of a mirror or with friends or family is another potential between-sessions activity.

Judith and Aaron Beck explain that without between-session assignments, treatment can't really be considered classic CBT, as homework reviews are crucial in the CBT session.

Popular CBT author David Burns acknowledges that it is not uncommon for clients to show resistance by not doing their homework. In his *Feeling Good Handbook*, he shares how he handled the resistance with one particular client. After his client came to session week after week without having done his homework, he used a bit of reverse psychology by suggesting that it didn't seem as if he was the right therapist for his client, as his approach incorporated homework, and apparently these expectations were not welcome by the client's consistent lack of follow-through. Burns suggested to his client that he could refer him to other therapists whose expectations of their clients were not as high, which might be a better fit for him. This proved to be a pivotal point in therapy, and the client began to work hard between sessions to complete the assignments.

Devising homework assignments at the end of the session is an important part of any solution-oriented approach.

☑ 6. Get in the Habit of Asking for Feedback

One of the hallmarks of the classic CBT session is to ask for feedback. Attempting to get feedback throughout the session is crucial to the solution-oriented approach. Judith Beck stresses the importance of watching for changes in facial expressions that would indicate anger, upset, anxiety, and so forth as a way of informally getting client feedback (J. S. Beck, 2011).

I often end the session with questions such as these: "What are your takeaways from the session today?" "Have we met your goals for the session?" (tying this in to goal clarification at the start of the session), and "How did you feel about what we talked about today?" By doing this, I am inviting them to tell me what they thought, how they felt, and if their goals for the session were met. I make sure to try to leave at least a few minutes for this type of wrap-up at the session's end. For some clients who are more reticent, I often leave the last ten minutes or so for a session review, as I have learned with some clients that my direct questioning at the end often leads to the most fruitful discussions.

By personally inviting feedback, I often get very valuable information as to how the client perceives what went on during the session. Much of the time our perceptions coincide, but sometimes I am surprised by how they processed the session. Some clients tend to misinterpret more than others, and for those clients I try to leave more time for feedback and clarification. One particular example that struck me occurred when I congratulated my client on doing so well and really making progress after months of treatment resistance. When I asked for her feedback at the end of the session, I found her response quite startling. She interpreted my compliments as a way for me to get rid of her as a client. Midway through the session, I had noticed that she became quieter, but did not realize the extent of her upset until I invited her feedback.

☑ 7. Use Metaphors to Unlock Emotion and Insight

As we have seen many times in the book, metaphors offer rich opportunities for therapeutic growth and healing. These are some of the reasons they are so powerful:

Metaphors . . .

Allow us to shift our perspective and unlock old ways of thinking
Help us think flexibly and in new ways
Encourage creativity in problem solving

Are one of the best solutions for treatment resistance

Evoke emotions and feelings that are key to change

Offer us increased insight by associating a concept with an example that we understand well in everyday life

Serve as reminders in clients' everyday lives that help keep them positive and reinforce the therapeutic concepts learned

We all use metaphors frequently in our daily lives and often don't even realize that we're doing it. So often, figures of speech are metaphors, and they are so well entrenched that we sometimes forget that they can't be taken literally. For example, "painting yourself into a corner" is an expression we all know, but it is not really about using paint. It refers to how *we are boxing ourselves in* (using another metaphor!)—or better yet *trapping* ourselves—making us a *prisoner* in the corner. You get the idea of how we use a *boatload* of metaphors all the time, and often do not even realize it! Can you think of others? Or do you want to just *cross that bridge* when you come to it?

☑ 8. Use Metaphorical Props

The metaphorical toolkits at the end of each chapter emphasize the importance of using actual metaphorical objects and props. There is something very powerful about stocking an office drawer with objects that your clients can carry with them or that you can use to trigger therapeutic lessons. While I am treating a client, I am constantly thinking of what metaphor would help them. I brainstorm with them what small article they can bring around in their purse or back pocket that will represent something soothing and helpful as they cope with challenges.

Some props can serve a variety of metaphorical lessons. An example of a very versatile and powerful prop is the finger trap mentioned in previous chapters. The trap demonstrates that the more you pull in a time of conflict, and the more you argue and try to prove you are right, the more you and the other person gets stuck. I love using this prop when working with argumentative couples in my office.

ACT founder Steven Hayes uses the finger trap to demonstrate the concept of acceptance. In his use of the metaphorical prop, he demonstrates his view that human pain and suffering results from trying to avoid and suppress feelings and thoughts rather than just letting them happen.

☑ 9. Use Role-Play Variations for Skill Building

Role-playing with clients gives them powerful and practical opportunities to practice skills learned in the session, especially when dealing with relationship issues that can be played out in the session. During a role play, I often use my communication handouts, such as "The Three Types of Communication" (Handout 6.2), as a basis for analyzing the level of assertive communication. We focus on using *I* statements instead of *you* statements.

Switching roles so that you play the role of your client and your client takes the role of a parent, spouse, or coworker can also be quite effective, as is switching the client and therapist roles so that you play the client and he or she plays the therapist. In working with groups, having clients pair up with one or two other people or work in small groups in which people take turns with their roles can be quite fun as well as enlightening. Role play allows clients to practice asserting themselves in situations that post challenges for them, and gives them ideas of how to handle difficult people in their lives. It's one thing to *talk about* how to handle situations, but another thing to *practice* it. Role play is one of the most effective therapeutic techniques I use in helping clients improve their self-esteem and interpersonal relationships.

Role play can also be a vehicle for enacting internal thoughts, thereby making them external. For example, you can play the client combatting the irrational thought monsters that keep speaking inside their heads. Externalizing these monsters and arguing against their aggressive statements can help clients stand up to their worst fears. This is the idea behind David Burns's Feared Fantasy technique, mentioned earlier in the book, as well as his technique of externalization of voices, in which the therapist or group members play out each other's positive and negative thoughts. In this case, a group member plays out another group member's irrational and negative thoughts, who in turn gets practice confronting those negative thoughts with more positive thoughts. With a group member acting out their own internal negative thoughts, individuals gain some skills and perspective to challenge them.

In sum, there is no end to the variations of role-playing that you can do with your client, and even if the situation would never happen in real life, it can certainly bring up real feelings and provide real learning that your clients can readily use outside the office.

☑ 10. Use Positive Psychology and Wellness Resources Online

Wellness solutions focused on work, school, and home, and balancing among them, are an outgrowth of the field of Positive Psychology. Psychologist Martin Seligman founded this psychological orientation in the last couple of decades. It was spearheaded at the University of Pennsylvania, and focuses on the empirical study of such things as positive emotions, strengths-based character, and healthy interpretations.

This focus on positive psychology, bundled with CBT and third-wave treatments, offers clients not only treatment solutions to problems but also wellness solutions for thriving—*not just surviving*.

Social media sites including blogs, inspirational posts on Facebook, and websites offering wellness tips are just some examples of Internet-based resources normalizing attention to mental health and wellness. Positive psychology has put wellness at the forefront of mainstream self-help, where the focus is on strengths, life satisfaction, and wellness instead of deficits and problems. With the wealth of resources available on the Internet, our clients can benefit from the many wellness and inspirational messages provided through blogs, mental health websites, Facebook, and Pinterest posts, to name just some of the avenues available on the web. In the resources section at the end of this chapter, I have included a few of my favorite wellness links. For example, self-help questionnaires like Ed Diener's famous Satisfaction With Life Scale offer quick and easy tools for growth and emotional well-being.

☑ 10 Ultimate Therapeutic Solutions Checklist

This checklist can serve as a reminder of practices to include in your solution-oriented therapy.

_____ 1. Use psychoeducation to teach clients in almost every session.
Strategy Note _____

_____

_____ 2. Start each session with a mood check.
Strategy Note _____

_____

_____ 3. Start each session by clarifying goals.
Strategy Note _____

_____

_____ 4. Use creative visualizations and experiential activities.
Strategy Note _____

_____

_____ 5. Use self-help assignments between sessions.
Strategy Note _____

_____

_____ 6. Get in the habit of asking for feedback.
Strategy Note _____

_____

_____ 7. Use metaphors to unlock emotion and insight.
Strategy Note _____

_____

_____ 8. Use metaphorical props.
Strategy Note _____

_____

_____ 9. Use role-play variations for skill building.
Strategy Note _____

_____ 10. Use positive psychology and wellness resources online.
Strategy Note _____

_____

Recommended Resources

Clinician Books

Cognitive Behavior Therapy: Basics and Beyond
  Judith S. Beck
Cognitive Therapy Techniques: A Practitioner's Guide
  Robert L. Leahy
Self-Help That Works: Resources to Improve Emotional Health and
  Strengthen Relationships
  John C. Norcross, Linda F. Campbell, John M. Grohol, John W. Santrock.
  Florin Selagea, and Robert Sommer
The CBT Toolbox: A Workbook for Clients and Clinicians
  Jeff Riggenbach
The Big Book of ACT Metaphors: A Practitioner's Guide to Experiential
  Exercises & Metaphors in Acceptance & Commitment Therapy
  Jill A. Stoddard and Niloofar Afari

Links

Association for Contextual Behavioral Science
"Acceptance & Commitment Therapy (ACT)" by Steven Hayes
  http://contextualscience.org/act
Beck Institute for Cognitive Behavior Therapy
(See especially Depression Inventory, Anxiety Inventory, and Hopeful-
  ness Scale)
  www.beckinstitute.org
  www.beckscales.com
Belmont Wellness: Emotional Wellness for Positive Living
(Psychoeducational client resources)
  http://www.belmontwellness.com/for-mental-health-professionals/
  psychoeducational-handouts-quizzes-group-activities/
David Burns: Feeling Good
  http://feelinggood.com
The Linehan Institute: Behavioral Tech
  http://behavioraltech.org

University of Illinois at Urbana-Champaign
Ed Diener
Satisfaction With Life Scale (SWLS)
  http://internal.psychology.illinois.edu/~ediener/SWLS.html
University of Pennsylvania, Positive Psychology Center
  http://www.ppc.sas.upenn.edu

Bibliography

Addis, M., Jacobson, M., & Martell, C. (2001). *Depression in context: Strategies for guided action.* New York, NY: Norton.

Alberti, R. E., & Emmons, M. L. (1990). *A manual for assertiveness trainers.* New York, NY: Impact.

Alberti, R. E., & Emmons, M. L. (2008). *Your perfect right: Assertiveness and equality in your life and relationships.* New York, NY: Impact.

Altman, D. (2014). *The mindfulness toolbox: 50 practical tips, tools & handouts for anxiety, depression, stress & pain.* Wisconsin: PESI.

American Psychological Association, American Institute of Stress. (2013). Stress statistics. Retrieved from http://www.statisticbrain.com/stress-statistics/

Anchor, S. (2010). *The happiness advantage: The seven principles of positive psychology that fuel success and performance at work.* New York, NY: Crown Business.

Anxiety and Depression Association of America. (n.d.). Facts & statistics. Retrieved August 14, 2014, from http://www.adaa.org/about-adaa/press-room/facts-statistics

Barker, P. (1985). *Using metaphors in psychotherapy.* New York, NY: Brunner/Mazel.

Beck, A. (1979). *Cognitive therapy and the emotional disorders.* New York, NY: Plume.

Beck, A., Rush, A., Shaw, B., & Emery, G. (1987). *Cognitive therapy of depression.* New York, NY: Guilford Press.

Beck, J. (2008). *The Beck diet solution: Train your brain to think like a thin person.* Alabama: Oxmoor House.

Beck, J. S. (2011). *Cognitive behavior therapy: Basics and beyond.* New York, NY: Guilford Press.

Belmont, J. A. (2006a). *86 TIPS (treatment ideas & practical strategies) for the therapeutic toolbox.* Wisconsin: PESI.

Belmont, J. A. (2006b). *The therapeutic toolbox: 103 group activities and treatment ideas & practical strategies.* Wisconsin: PESI.

Belmont, J. A. (2007). *The therapeutic companion: Tips to increase your mental fitness.* Pennsylvania: Worksite Insights.

Belmont, J. A. (2013). *127 more amazing tips and tools for the therapeutic toolbox.* Wisconsin: PESI.

Belmont, J. A., & Shor, L. (2012). *The Swiss cheese theory of life: How to get through life's holes without getting stuck in them!* Wisconsin: Premier/ PESI.

Benson, H., with Klipper, M. (1975). *The relaxation response.* New York, NY: William Morrow.

Bloom, L., Coburn, K., & Pearlman, J. (1977). *The new assertive woman.* New York, NY: Dell.

Bourne, E. J. (1990). *The anxiety and phobia workbook.* California: New Harbinger.

Burdick, D. (2013). *Mindfulness skills workbook for clinicians & clients: 111 tools, techniques, activities & worksheets.* Wisconsin: PESI.

Burns, D. D. (1980). *Feeling good: The new mood therapy.* New York, NY: HarperCollins.

Burns, D. D. (1993a). *Ten days to self-esteem.* New York, NY: HarperCollins.

Burns, D. D. (1993b). *Ten days to self-esteem: The leader's manual.* New York, NY: Quill William Morrow.

Burns, D. D. (1999). *The feeling good handbook.* New York, NY: Penguin Group.

Burns, D. D. (2006). *When panic attacks: The new, drug-free anxiety therapy that can change your life.* New York, NY: Three Rivers Press.

Byock, I. (2004). *The four things that matter most: A book about living.* New York, NY: Simon & Schuster.

Carnegie, D. (1948). *How to stop worrying and start living.* New York, NY: Simon & Schuster.

Carter, L., & Minirth, F. (1997). *The choosing to forgive workbook*. Tennessee: Thomas Nelson.

Clark, D. A., & Beck, A. T. (2011). *The anxiety and worry workbook: The cognitive behavioral solution*. New York, NY: Guilford Press.

Culver, L., McKinney, B., & Paradise, L. (2011). *Mental health professionals' experiences of vicarious traumatization in post–Hurricane Katrina New Orleans.*

Curran, L. A. (2013). *101 trauma-informed interventions*. Wisconsin: Premier.

Diener, E. (2009). *Assessing well-being: The collected works of Ed Diener* (Social Indicators Research Series). New York, NY: Springer.

Dimeff, L., & Linehan, M. (2001). Dialectical behavior therapy in a nutshell. *The California Psychologist, 34,* 10–13

Doran, G. T. (1981). "There's a S.M.A.R.T. way to write management's goals and objectives." *Management Review* (AMA FORUM) 70(11): 35–36.

Eifert, G. H., & Forsyth, J. P. (2005a). *Acceptance & commitment therapy for anxiety disorders: A practitioner's treatment guide to using mindfulness, acceptance, and values-based behavior change strategies*. California: New Harbinger.

Eifert, G. H., & Forsyth, J. P. (2005b) *Acceptance and commitment therapy for anxiety disorders: Three case studies exemplifying a unified treatment protocol*. California: New Harbinger.

Eifert, G. H., McKay, M., Forsyth, J. P., & Hayes, S. (2006). *ACT on life not on anger: The new Acceptance and Commitment Therapy guide to problem anger*. California: New Harbinger.

Ellis, A. (1998). *How to control your anxiety before it controls you*. New York, NY: Kensington.

Ellis, A., & Harper, R. A. (1975). *A new guide to rational living*. New Jersey: Prentice Hall.

Ellis, A., & MacLaren, C. (2005). *Rational emotive behavior therapy: A therapist's guide*. California: Impact.

Fanning, P., & McKay, M., (2008). *Progressive relaxation* (Relaxation & Stress Reduction) [Audiobook, CD]. California: New Harbinger.

Ferster, C. (1973, October). A functional analysis of depression. *American Psychologist,* pp. 857–870.

Figley, C. R. (1995). *Compassion fatigue as secondary stress disorder: An overview. Compassion fatigue: Coping with secondary traumatic stress disorder in those who treat the traumatized.* New York, NY: Brunner/Mazel.

Fox, D. J. (2014). *Diagnosis & treatment of personality disorders.* Wisconsin: PESI.

Fralich, T. (2013). *The five core skills of mindfulness: A direct path to more confidence, joy and love.* Wisconsin: PESI.

Frankel, E. (2003). *Sacred therapy: Jewish spiritual teachings on emotional healing and inner wholeness.* Boston, MA: Shambhala Press.

Freeman, A. (1989). *Woulda, coulda, shoulda: Overcoming regrets, mistakes, and missed opportunities.* New York, NY: HarperCollins.

Friedman, M. (1996). *Type A behavior: Its diagnosis and treatment.* New York, NY: Plenum Press (Kluwer Academic Press).

Friedman, M., & Rosenman, R. (1959). Association of specific overt behavior pattern with blood and cardiovascular findings. *Journal of the American Medical Association, 169*(12), 1286–1296.

Gregory, B. (2010). *Cognitive-behavioral therapy skills workbook.* Wisconsin: Premier.

Harris, R. (2009). *ACT made simple: An easy-to-read primer on Acceptance and Commitment Therapy.* California: New Harbinger.

Hayes, S. C. (2005). *Get out of your mind & into your life: The new acceptance & commitment therapy.* California: New Harbinger.

Hayes, S. C., Strosahl, K. D., & Wilson, K. G. (1999) *Acceptance and commitment therapy.* New York, NY: Guilford Press.

Henderson, L. (2014). *Helping your shy and socially anxious client: A social fitness training protocol using CBT.* California: New Harbinger.

Hibbs, S. (2013). *Anxiety treatment techniques that really work.* Wisconsin: Premier.

Jacobson, N. S., Dobson, K. S., Truax, P. A., Addis, M. E., Koerner, K., Gollan, J. K. . . . Prince, S. E. (1996). A component analysis of cognitive-behavioral treatment for depression. *Journal of Consulting and Clinical Psychology, 64,* 295–304.

Jones, A. (1998). *104 activities that build: Self-esteem, teamwork, communi-cation, anger management, self-discovery, coping skills.* Maryland: Rec Room.

Kabat-Zinn, J. (2005). *Guided mindfulness meditation (Book 1).* Colorado: Sounds True.

Kabat-Zinn, J. (2012a). *Guided mindfulness meditation (Book 3).* Colorado: Sounds True.

Kabat-Zinn, J. (2012b). *Mindfulness for beginners.* Colorado: Sounds True.

Kabat-Zinn, J. (2014). *Guided mindfulness meditation (Book 2).* Colorado: Sounds True.

Kassinove, H., & Tafrate, R. C. (2002) *Anger management: The complete treatment guidebook for practitioners.* California: Impact.

Knaus, W. J. (2012). *The cognitive behavioral workbook for depression.* California: New Harbinger.

Kobasa, S. C. (1979). Stressful life events, personality and health: Inquiry into hardiness. *Journal of Personality and Social Psychology, 37*(1): 1–11.

Kopp, R. (1995). *Metaphor therapy: Using client generated metaphors in psychotherapy.* New York, NY: Brunner/Mazel.

Kubler-Ross, E. (1969). *On death and dying.* New York, NY: Scribner.

Lawler, K., Younger, J. W., Piferi, R. L., Billington, E., Jobe, R., Edmond-son, K., & Jones, W. H. (2003). A change of heart: Cardiovascular correlates of forgiveness in response to interpersonal conflict. Journal of Behavioral Medicine, 26(5), 373–393.

Lawler, K., Younger, J. W., Piferi, R. L., Jobe, R. L., Edmondson, K, A., & Jones, W. H. (2005). The unique effects of forgiveness on health: An exploration of pathways. *Journal of Behavioral Medicine, 28*(2), 157–167.

Leahy, R. L. (2003). *Cognitive therapy techniques: A practitioner's guide.* New York, NY: Guilford Press.

Linehan, M. M. (1993). *Skills training manual for treating borderline per-sonality disorder.* New York, NY: Guilford Press.

Luskin, F. (2003). *Forgive for good: A proven prescription for health and happiness.* New York, NY: HarperOne.

Lyddon, W. J., Clay, A. L., & Sparks, C. L. (2001). Metaphor and change in counseling. *Journal of Counseling and Development, 79,* 269–274.

Madders, J. (1997). *The stress and relaxation handbook: A practical guide to self-help techniques.* London, UK: Vermilion.

Marra, T. (2005). *Dialectical behavior therapy in private practice: A practical & comprehensive guide.* California: New Harbinger.

Mayo Clinic Staff. (2011, November 23). Forgiveness: Letting go of grudges and bitterness. Retrieved from http://www.mayoclinic.org /healthy-living/adult-health/in-depth/forgiveness/art-20047692

McKay, M., Davis, M., & Fanning, P. (2007). *Thoughts & feelings: Taking control of your moods & your life.* California: New Harbinger.

McKay, M., Lev, A., & Skeen, M. (2012). *Acceptance and commitment therapy for interpersonal problems.* California: New Harbinger.

McKay, M., & Rogers, P. (2007). *The anger control workbook.* California: New Harbinger.

McKay, M., Rogers, P. D., & McKay, J. (2003). *When anger hurts: Quieting the storm within.* California: New Harbinger.

McKay, M., & Wood, J. (2011). *The Dialectical Behavior Therapy diary.* California: New Harbinger.

McKay, M., Wood, J. C., & Brantley, J. (2007). *The Dialectical Behavior Therapy skills workbook: Practical DBT exercises for learning mindfulness, interpersonal effectiveness, emotion regulation & tolerance.* California: New Harbinger.

Miller, W., & Rollnick, S. (2012). *Motivational interviewing: Helping people change* (3rd ed.). New York, NY: Guilford Press.

Nolen-Hoekesema, S. (2004). *Women who think too much: How to break free of overthinking and reclaim your life.* New York, NY: Henry Holt.

Norcross, J. C., Campbell, L. F., Grohol, J. M., Santrock, J. W., Selagea, F., & Sommer, R. (2013). *Self-help that works: Resources to improve emotional health and strengthen relationships.* New York, NY: Oxford University Press.

Pollak, S. M., Pedulla, T., & Siegel, R. D. (2014). *Sitting together: Essential skills for mindfulness-based psychotherapy.* New York, NY: Guilford Press.

Prochaska, J. O., Norcross, J. C., & DiClemente, C. C. (1994). *Changing for good.* New York, NY: Morrow.

Riggenbach, J. (2013). *The CBT toolbox: A workbook for clients and clinicians.* Wisconsin: Premier.

Rizzo, T. H. (2006, September). The healing power of forgiveness. *IDEA Fitness Journal.* Retrieved from http://www.ideafit.com/fitness-library/healing-power-forgiveness

Roese, N. (2005). *If only: How to turn regret into opportunity.* New York, NY: Random House.

Rogers, C.R. (1959). A theory of therapy, personality, and interpersonal relationships as developed in the client-centered framework. Reprinted in H. Kirschenbaum and V. Henderson (Eds.) *The Carl Rogers Reader* (1989). Boston: Houghton Mifflin.

Roth, G. (1991). *When food is love.* New York, NY, Penguin Books.

Salcedo, B. (2007). *Progressive muscle relaxation: 20 minutes to total relaxation [Single]*

Schiraldi, G. R. (2001). *The self-esteem workbook.* California: New Harbinger.

Schiraldi, G. R. (2007). *10 simple solutions for building self-esteem: How to end self-doubt, gain confidence, & create a positive self-image.* California: New Harbinger.

Seaward, B. L. (2011). *Health and wellness journal workbook.* Massachusetts: Jones & Bartlett.

Seaward, B. L. (2014). *Essentials of managing stress.* Massachusetts: Jones & Bartlett.

Segal, Z. V., Williams, J. M., & Teasdale, J. D. (2001). *Mindfulness-based cognitive therapy for depression: A new approach to preventing relapse.* New York, NY: Guilford Press.

Segal, Z. V., Williams, J. M. G., & Teasdale, J. D. (2013). *Mindfulness-based cognitive therapy for depression.* New York, NY: Guilford Press.

Seligman, M. (2007). *The optimistic child: A proven program to safeguard children against depression and build lifelong resilience.* New York, NY: Houghton Mifflin.

Selye, H. (1979). *Self-help for your anxiety: How to eliminate fear and stress from your life.* New York, NY: Barnes & Noble.

Selye, H. (1974). *Stress Without Distress.* Philadelphia, PA: Lippincott Williams & Wilkins.

Shapiro, R. (2010). *Goodbye worries: Guided meditation to train your mind to quiet your thoughts.* Roberta Shapiro Productions.

Sharpe, R. (1979). *Self-help for your anxiety: How to eliminate fear and stress from your life.* New York, NY: Barnes & Noble.

Simon, S. B., & Simon, S. (2007). *Forgiveness: How to make peace with your past and get on with your life.* New York, NY: Grand Central.

Smedes, L. B. (2007). *Forgive and forget: Healing the hurts we don't deserve.* New York, NY: HarperOne.

Sobel, D., & Ornstein, R. (1996). *The healthy mind, healthy body handbook.* Los Altos, CA: DRx.

Somov, P. G. (2013). *Anger management jumpstart: A 4-session mindfulness path to compassion and change.* Wisconsin: PESI.

Stoddard, J. A., & Afari, N. (2014). *The big book of ACT metaphors: A practitioner's guide to experiential exercises and metaphors in Acceptance and Commitment Therapy.* California: New Harbinger.

Teasdale, J., Williams, M., & Segal, Z. (2014). *The mindful way workbook.* New York, NY: Guilford Press.

Toussaint, L., Owen, A. D., & Cheadle, A. (2012). Forgive to live: Forgiveness, health, and longevity. *Journal of Behavioral Medicine, 35*(4), 375–386.

Van Dijk, S. (2012). *DBT made simple: A step-by-step guide to Dialectical Behavior Therapy.* California: New Harbinger.

Viorst, J. (1986). *Necessary losses: The loves, illusions, dependencies, and impossible expectations that all of us have to give up in order to grow.* New York, NY: Fireside.

Virtue, D. (1998). *Chakra cleaning.* California: Hay House.

Wolpe, J. (1968). *Psychotherapy by reciprocal inhibition.* New York, NY: Springer-Verlag.

Wolpe, J. (1973). *The practice of behavior therapy.* New York, NY: Pergamon Press.

Index